The Pathology of the Carotid Body and Sinus

The Pathology of the Carotid Body and Sinus

Donald Heath
MD (Sheffield), DSc (Sheffield), PhD (Birmingham), FRCP, FRCPath

George Holt Professor of Pathology, University of Liverpool;
Honorary Consultant in Pathology, Royal Liverpool Hospital

Paul Smith
BSc, PhD (Liverpool)

Senior Lecturer in Pathology, University of Liverpool

Edward Arnold

First published in Great Britain 1985 by
Edward Arnold (Publishers) Ltd, 41 Bedford Square, London WC1B 3DQ

Edward Arnold (Australia) Pty Ltd, 80 Waverley Road, Caulfield East, Victoria 3145, Australia

British Library Cataloguing in Publication Data

Heath, Donald
The pathology of the carotid body and sinus.
1. Carotid gland — Diseases
I. Title II. Smith, Paul
616.8 RC936

ISBN 0-7131-4466-1

Text set in 10/12 Plantin by
CK Typesetters, 26 Mulgrave Road,
Sutton, Surrey
Printed in Great Britain by
Butler & Tanner Ltd, Frome and London

Preface

The carotid body is the forgotten organ of morbid anatomy. Although it has been recognized as a chemoreceptor for over half a century and appears to be closely linked with the function of baroreception, it is rarely examined at necropsy by the pathologist even in cases of heart and lung disease where changes in the carotid body might be anticipated. As a result a peculiar imbalance has developed over our knowledge of the carotid body. Physiologists carry out elegant experiments in various species of animal and continue to argue over the mechanism of chemoreception and the identity of its transducer. Pathologists ignore the carotid body and remain uninformed about the alterations in glomic tissue in various generalized diseases. This small book is an attempt to begin to remedy this unsatisfactory state of affairs. It is meant to introduce morbid anatomists to what is known about the pathology of the human carotid body and sinus. It has been written primarily for the practising pathologist rather than the neurophysiologist and is concerned, wherever possible, with human rather than animal tissues. At present much of what we know about the pathology of glomic tissue is controversial and speculative but, if this book encourages pathologists to start taking an interest in the carotid body, much will have been achieved and progress in our understanding of this organ could be anticipated.

We wish to thank Miss Linda Byron for her patience with the typing of the manuscript and Mr Alan Williams for his photographic skill in the preparation of the illustrations.

Donald Heath
Paul Smith
Liverpool 1985

Contents

1. The Nature of the Carotid Body

Situated at the bifurcation of the common carotid artery on both sides of the neck is a complex arrangement of blood vessels, nerves and cells which monitors vital physiological functions. Blood may flow past the bifurcation into the internal carotid artery to supply the brain and other structures. The origin of this vessel shows abrupt thinning of its media, often with some dilatation, to form the *carotid sinus* which functions as a baroreceptor (Figs 1.1 and 1.2) (Chapter 12). Alternatively it may flow into the external carotid artery to supply the face and other tissues. A third stream enters the minute but important glomic arteries, one or more on both sides, which may arise from the carotid bifurcation itself or from the first part of the external carotid artery (Fig. 1.1). The glomic arteries run to supply the *carotid body* which is a small organ situated in the fork of the bifurcation (Figs 1.1 and 1.2). This nodule of tissue is known to be a chemoreceptor but it also appears to be directly sensitive to the level of intravascular pressure (Chapter 8). It may well be that the carotid body has other as yet undiscovered functions, perhaps related to its secretion of a peptide hormone. At present, understanding of the physiology of the carotid body is incomplete and controversial, and knowledge of its pathology even more so.

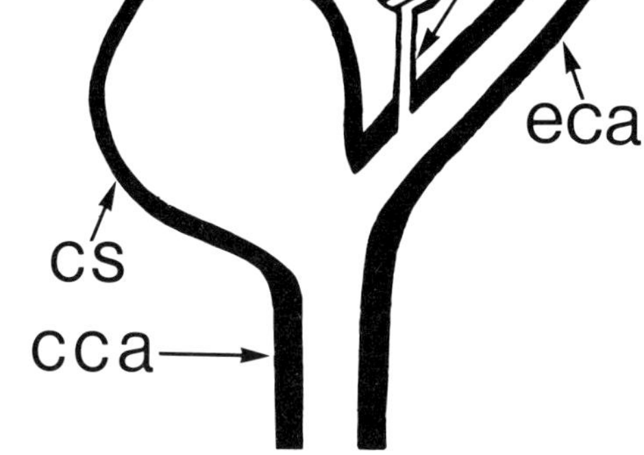

Fig. 1.1 Diagram to illustrate the vascular connections of the carotid body and sinus. The common carotid artery (cca) divides into internal (ica) and external (eca) branches. The first part of the internal carotid artery is dilated to form the carotid sinus (cs) subserving baroreception. The carotid body (cb), whose major function is generally accepted to be chemoreception, is supplied by blood through one or more glomic arteries (ga) which commonly arise from the the external carotid artery.

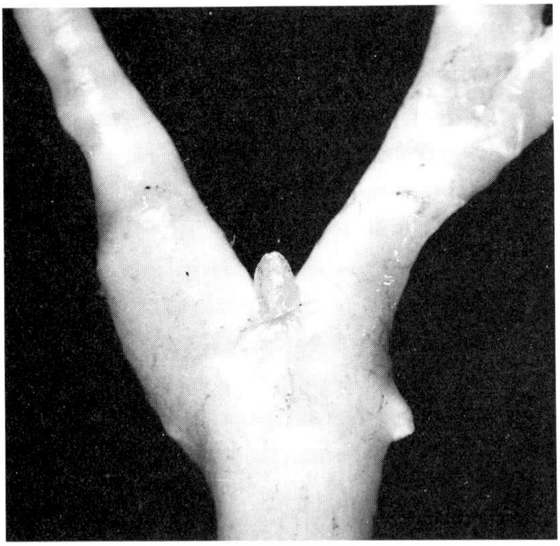

Fig. 1.2 Left carotid bifurcation from a woman of 21 years who died from Goodpasture's syndrome. The carotid sinus and body are recognized with ease on comparison with the previous figure. The left carotid body weighed 3.7 mg. (× 3.4)

Hence it is essential to keep an open mind as to the functions of the carotid body and its behaviour in disease.

Discovery of the carotid body

In 1742 Haller demonstrated nerve twigs leaving what he considered to be a small hitherto undescribed ganglion in the carotid bifurcation (Adams, 1958). This discovery of a 'ganglion minutum' was referred to by both of his pupils, Taube and Berckelman, in their inaugural dissertations in the following two years. Their reports were republished by Haller in his 'Disputationum Anatomicarum' in 1747 and 1749. In 1797 there was a posthumous publication by Andersch, an ex-pupil of Haller, who died in 1777 and who claimed to have been the first to see the carotid body, giving an accurate account of its blood supply. In 1772 Neubauer working independently of Haller and his group, also published an illustrated account of the carotid body and its nerve supply. Mayer (1833) was of the opinion that Haller and his pupils had described an inconstant ganglion of the cervical sympathetic chain and he provided himself what he considered to be the first description of the carotid body. He noted that the carotid body was attached to the wall of the carotid bifurcation by a ligamentous strand of tissue. It is now known that this strand encloses the glomic artery carrying the blood supply to the carotid body and it is called to this day 'Mayer's ligament'.

The nature of the carotid body

Thus, by 1833, the stage was set for further investigation by anatomists, embryologists, physiologists and pathologists. Since that time the carotid body has been studied intensively but in spite of this its nature remains controversial.

Early on it was appreciated that the carotid body is composed of three main elements. There is a parenchyma of cells of two types, one being large and round and the other slender and elongated. This is framed around a rich plexus of arteries, capillaries and veins. A profuse nerve network supplies both the vascular and parenchymal elements. These integral parts of the carotid body have to be taken into account when considering the nature of the carotid body, and the nomenclature used to describe it. Decisions on its nature in their turn determine the proper setting in which its pathology should be considered.

Glomus and glomic tissue

One of the most characteristic features of the carotid body is the complex network of arteries, capillaries and veins that make it into a highly vascular ball of tissue. The Latin word for a rolled-up body or ball is '*glomus*' and this term is classically used in descriptive histology to indicate a spherical conglomeration of cells and small vessels. Thus, in its diminutive form, it is used to describe the renal glomerulus. Care must be taken not to confuse the term 'glomus' in this sense with the glomus found in the subcutaneous tissue of the fingers and toes. The cutaneous glomus represents a collection of arteriovenous anastomoses and, as we shall see in Chapter 9, such vascular connections are not a feature of the human carotid body. Hence, throughout this book, we shall use the terms glomus and glomic tissue in a non-specific sense merely implying a sphere of vascular tissue exhibiting an intimate association of cells and small blood vessels.

The basic histological unit

The cellular parenchyma of the carotid body consists of two types of cell. One has a large round nucleus and copius cytoplasm containing vesicles rich in biogenic amines; it is termed the chief cell. The other is an elongated slender cell closely wrapped around nerve axons; it is thus called the sheath, supporting or sustentacular cell. These cells are commonly arranged in clusters, the chief cells in the centre and the sustentacular cells at the periphery. In the connective tissue between clusters there are Schwann cells which are very similar in appearance to sustentacular cells. A third elongated cell, the pericyte, is seen arranged circumferentially around small blood vessels.

The carotid body is not alone in showing this basic histological structure. There are glomera widely scattered throughout the body consisting of a highly vascular tissue intimately admixed with a cellular parenchyma composed of rounded chief cells and elongated sustentacular cells. Following a most meticulous study of the glomera in fetuses, Kjaergaard (1973) concluded that there is no histological or ultrastructural criterion by which the carotid body can be distingushed from other glomera and thus it appears to be part of a generalized system. Glenner and Grimley (1974) believe that the histological similarities are sufficient to merit grouping together several neoplasms which occur in widely separated sites in the body and we shall note examples of them in

Chapter 10. They consider that the glomera fall into the four following groups but it is prudent to bear in mind that similarity in histological appearance does not necessarily imply that the tissues have the same function.

Branchiomeric

This is the group which includes the carotid body. A word of explanation is necessary concerning this term 'branchiomeric'. As long as it was believed that the glomera were derived from the mesoderm in the baroreceptive vascular zones, that is that they were derived from cells in the branchial arches, they were termed branchiogenic. An extremely intimate connection between the glomera and the respective vascular zone had to be presupposed (Kjaergaard, 1973). Later it was discovered that the glomera were *branchiomeric*, that is, *laid down* at the site of the branchial arches. They were thought to be derived from cells, be they neurectodermal or ectodermal, which migrate along the nerves corresponding to the branchial arches. Thus, for example, the migration may be along the glossopharyngeal nerve to the third branchial arch. Thus, it would appear that the nervous connections predominate over the vascular.

This group also includes jugulotympanic glomic tissue in the adventitia of the bulb of the jugular vein immediately beneath the bony floor of the middle ear or along the tympanic branch of the glossopharyngeal nerve. This was described by Guild (1941) as the 'glomus jugularis' (properly 'glomus jugulare'). Others are the aortico-pulmonary bodies which have been described just above the ductus arteriosus in the angle between this vessel and the descending portion of the arch of the aorta, near the root of the innominate artery, on the anterolateral aspect of the left part of the aortic arch, and near the origin of the left coronary artery. One of these nodules is found on the bifurcation of the pulmonary trunk where it has acquired the spurious designation of the 'glomus pulmonale' (Chapter 11). Orbital glomera have been described in both man and the chimpanzee. Laryngeal glomera have been described just above the anterior end of the vocal cords and between the thyroid and cricoid cartilages (Glenner and Grimley, 1974).

Intravagal

Groups of glomic cells are found interior to the perineurium just beneath the nerve sheath or between nerve fibres (Glenner and Grimley, 1974). Such glomera have been described within or below the ganglion nodosum of the vagus nerve where it is termed the 'glomus intravagale'. Such glomera are not related to arteries but cannot be distinguished from other glomic tissue on grounds of histology, ultrastructure or cytochemistry.

Aortico-sympathetic

These are associated with segmental ganglia of the sympathetic chain and collateral ganglia. A member of this group, especially prominent in the fetus and newborn is the organ of Zuckerkandl.

Visceral-autonomic

These are associated with the blood vessels of viscera. One prominent group is found around pulmonary venules and we consider it further in Chapter 11. Other examples have been reported in the interatrial septum of the heart, in the hilus of the liver, in the wall of the urinary bladder and in association with the mesenteric vessels. Cell groups in association with the duodenal wall have been considered as further candidates for inclusion in this group.

Chromaffin paraganglia

At the turn of the century Kohn (1900) developed the concept that the carotid body and the system of glomera shared with the adrenal medulla the characteristic of staining with potassium dichromate and formed a system of chromaffin paraganglia. However, to classify glomera as paraganglia they have to meet certain strict criteria. Thus, the glomic cells must be homologous to the postganglionic sympathetic ganglion cells, their main innervation must be sympathetic efferent nerve fibres, the cells must secrete catecholamines, and they must be chromaffin (Kjaergaard, 1973). These criteria are not met by the glomera which cannot thus legitimately be regarded as chromaffin paraganglia.

Non-chromaffin paraganglia

The concept of the carotid body as a chromaffin paraganglion was discarded largely because glomic tissue was found to be non-chromaffin except to a minute degree (Chapter 3). To meet this objection Watzka (1930–31) introduced the concept of 'non-chromaffin paranganglia', as the parasympathetic homologue of the chromaffin paraganglia. The strict criteria to be met here are that the cells must be homologous to the postganglionic parasympathetic ganglion cells, their main innervation must be parasympathetic efferent nerve fibres, the cells must secrete an acetyl choline-like substance and the cells must be non-chromaffin (Kjaergaard, 1973). These criteria once again are not met by the glomera. Kjaergaard believes that the term paraganglion should be restricted to phaeochromocytes.

While the carotid body and the other glomera clearly cannot be regarded as parangangla this does not invalidate the concept that they constitute a well-defined system of tissues throughout the body. The appropriate designation for it will have to await further information on the physiology and pathology of its components. Throughout this book we shall employ the non-specific and non-committal term of 'glomic tissue'.

The carotid body as an endocrine gland

The first microscopic study of the carotid glomus was performed in 1862 by Luschka who thought that on histological grounds it was a gland. He assumed that it had developed from the pharyngeal epithelium and this view appeared to be supported by the studies of Stieda (1881) until Jacoby (1896) showed that Stieda had confused the primordium of glomic tissue with that of the inferior parathyroid gland. Luschka's concept of the carotid body as an endocrine gland of endodermal derivation seemed to be dead. However, the recent concept of Pearse (1969) of the APUD cell as one having the capacity for the formation, storage and secretion of peptides of low molecular weight has revived interest in old ideas. The dense osmiophilic cores of the neurosecretory vesicles (Chapter 4) may be composed of a peptide, called 'glomin', a suitably non-committal term, by Pearse. Recent studies by Wharton *et al.* (1980) have demonstrated neuropeptides in the carotid body of the cat. Enkephalin-like material occurred in considerable quantities in extracts of the organ and enkephalin-like immunoreactivity was localised in chief cells. Both vasoactive intestinal polypeptide and substance P-like immunoreactivity was also present but was localised in nerve fibres distributed throughout the organ.

The nerve network

The clusters of chief and sustentacular cells are supplied by a luxuriant nerve network. The general pathologist, used to the section stained by haematoxylin and eosin, must constantly bear in mind that the histological subjects he sees are enmeshed by numerous nerve filaments. These will become apparent only when he applies the staining techniques advocated in Chapter 3.

The carotid body receives its nerve supply from the glossopharyngeal (ninth cranial) nerve, through the carotid sinus nerve, and from the superior cervical sympathetic ganglion of the autonomic nervous system, through the ganglio-glomerular nerve. Kohn (1900) had assumed that the glomic cells of the carotid body were supplied by axons of sympathetic nerves. In 1926 de Castro cut the glossopharyngeal nerve at the point it emerged from the skull and found that the nerve subsequently degenerated. He assumed that these nerve fibres were a direct motor pathway from the brain stem and had a secretory function. Two years later in another experiment he cut the nerve intracranially and this time there was no degeneration. Clearly on this occasion the section had been made central to the sensory petrosal ganglion of the glossopharyngeal nerve. This led him to change his ground and to deduce that the ganglion was composed of sensory ganglion cells, and that the carotid body was a sensory organ, the glomus cells being receptor cells which initiated activity of adjacent sensory nerves. At the same time de Castro presented his brilliant intuitative interpretation of the histology of the carotid body as that of a chemoreceptor. This was soon confirmed physiologically (Heymans *et al.*, 1930).

Following on a report by Lever *et al.*, (1959) that nerve endings next to glomus cells contained numerous microvesicles, further work employing electron microscopy to study degeneration of nerve axons was carried out. A controversial paper was published by Biscoe and his associates (1970). They found fewer nerve endings on glomus cells after section of the glossopharyngeal nerve central to the sensory petrosal ganglion. They concluded that the vesicle-containing nerve endings on the glomus cells were efferent, thus reviving the original ideas of de Castro in 1926. Most have been unable to confirm this work and would still accept that most vesicle-containing nerve endings are part of unipolar neurons whose cell bodies are in the petrosal ganglion. Nevertheless, the possibility of motor effector nerve endings has to be kept in mind. Conceivably such nerve endings could instruct the carotid body to release peptide hormones from the dense cores of the vesicles of glomic chief cells as referred to above.

A few autonomic ganglion cells occur individually or in small groups near the periphery of the carotid body near its connections with the ganglioglomerular nerve. Both sympathetic and parasympathetic ganglion cells appear to be present, the former being innervated by sympathetic nerves and the latter by the glossopharyngeal nerve. They are large being between 20μm and 40μm in diameter. It seems likely that the ganglion cells are concerned with the innervation of the blood vessels of the carotid body, the sympathetic nerves causing vasoconstriction and the parasympathetic vasodilatation. As early as 1925 Drüner had proposed that the carotid body contained baroreceptors which, when stimulated, induced a reflex slowing of the heart. De Castro (1926) noted that nerve endings similar in structure to those in the carotid sinus were present on arteries and arterioles in the carotid body. These nerves come from myelinated axons of both the glossopharyngeal and vagus nerves.

There is evidence that in the cat at least some unmyelinated axons end in an envelopment of sustentacular cells without making contact with glomus cells (de Kock, 1951; de Kock and Dunn, 1966). In this connection it is of interest to note that Zapata and his colleagues (1976, 1977) crushed the carotid sinus nerve of cats and then studied changes in structure and function of the carotid body during regeneration. They found that the responsiveness of chemoreceptors to asphyxia and cyanide returned to normal as soon as six days after the nerve was crushed. Comparatively few axons were in contact with chief cells at that time. This suggests that regrowth of nerves to clusters (Chapter 3) is necessary for chemoreception but apposition of specialized nerve endings and glomus cells is not.

The axons next to glomus cells are fine unmyelinated fibres, with fusiform, triangular or calyx-shaped varicosities along their length, which end in small boutons or calyces which cover a bigger area of plasma membrane. The calyces and most boutons are sensory endings. Hence, size and shape are not reliable criteria for distinguishing sensory from motor nerve endings. Similarly, while small clear-cored vesicles are a prominent feature of motor nerve endings they are also pronounced in sensory nerve endings in the carotid body. Conditions which increase chemoreceptor activity decrease the number of vesicles. It is conceivable that the clear-core vesicles contain acetyl choline in contrast to the catecholamines and protein of dense-core vesicles.

In addition to the connections between nerve endings and cell there are numerous chemical synapses which are functional contacts between two neurons or between neurons and effector cells (McDonald, 1981). At these specialized synaptic junctions there are cytoplasmic densities which are attached asymmetrically to the cell membranes of the two cells which are themselves not thickened. On the presynaptic membrane these densities comprise dense projections but on the postsynaptic membrane the cytoplasmic density is not so condensed. Synaptic vesicles are present on the presynaptic side of the synaptic cleft 15–30 nm wide.

In summary, the picture that emerges of the innervation of the carotid body is one of complex neural circuits and chemical synapses. In the studies of McDonald and Mitchell (1975) on the rat carotid body most of the nerve terminals in contact with chief cells are from sensory axons which run in the carotid sinus nerve into the glossopharyngeal nerve and thence into its sensory petrosal ganglion wherein lie the cell bodies. They presumably transmit the stimuli concerned with chemoreception. A few effector nerve filaments reach the chief cells but their function is unknown. These glomus cells are in elaborate communication with one another by chemical synapses. The carotid sinus nerve also carries within it pre-ganglionic parasympathetic axons which connect with parasympathetic ganglion cells. The latter send effector nerves to blood vessels in the carotid body. Pre-ganglionic sympathetic axons enter through the ganglioglomerular nerve to reach sympathetic ganglion cells. These also send effector nerves to the blood vessels. Nerve axons leave the blood vessels to reach the ganglioglomerular nerve, perhaps concerned with baroreception. A few preganglionic sympathetic axons pass from the ganglioglomerular nerve direct to the glomus cells. Finally, it has to be kept in mind that some free, unmyelinated nerve axons appear to end in an envelopment by sustentacular cells.

Bioamines and peptides in chief cells

The chief cells described in Chapter 3 contain several potent compounds in their dense-core vesicles which are almost certainly concerned with the process of chemoreception. Prominent among these are the catecholamines. In a series of 76 pairs of carotid bodies removed at necropsy the percentage of four bioamines present were as follows: dopamine (3, 4 dihydroxyphenylethylamine) 64, serotonin (5, 6 hydroxytryptamine) 18.8, noradrenaline 14.8, and adrenaline 2.5 (Steele and Hinterberger, 1972). The concentration of dopamine in the carotid body is 20–40 μg/g while that of noradrenaline is only 1.5 μg/g (Dearnaley *et al.*, 1968). This predominance of dopamine over noradrenaline occurs in only one other area of the body, namely the corpus striatum and substantia nigra in the brain. While Steele and Hinterberger (1972) were able to demonstrate some association between high levels of dopamine in the carotid bodies and cerebrovascular disease, and to suggest a possible rôle of high carotid body serotonin content in some forms of systemic hypertension, they were unable to find any disturbance in the relative contents of the biogenic amines in subjects dying in respiratory failure with sustained chronic hypoxaemia.

Protein is a principal constituent of the core material of neurosecretory vesicles. Immunocytochemistry and radioimmunoassay have detected peptides related to the opiates such as enkephalin, substance P, and VIP-like peptides in the carotid body in the cat (Wharton *et al.,* 1980). The rôle of peptides and of the hypothetical hormone, 'glomin', from the carotid body is unknown.

Catecholamines and carotid body function

It might be anticipated that the carotid body has a local humoral function, releasing the bioamines to stimulate adjacent nerve terminals. Lever *et al.*, (1959) and Grimley and Glenner (1968) advanced this view, visualizing a local build up of neurotransmitter substances around sensory afferent nerves leading to depolarization of sensory fibres with the formation of impulse in the carotid sinus nerve. However, Eyzaguirre and Koyano (1965) found no increase in the frequency of electric discharges in the sinus nerve after the application of serotonin, adrenaline or noradrenaline. It was clear that the concept of a straightforward stimulatory rôle for released bioamines from chief cells was suspect. Furthermore, Blümcke *et al.*, (1967) believed that acetyl choline was in some way a transmitter for physiological stimuli in the process.

In 1975 Osborne and Butler suggested that secretion of dopamine from chief cells acts as an inhibitory transmitter. Under eupoxic conditions the dopamine may hyperpolarize the nerve endings thus reducing the spontaneous discharge frequency. Under conditions of hypoxia, the release of dopamine from chief cells is thought to be reduced, allowing the nerve endings to return to their depolarized state. Osborne and Butler thought that the depolarization might cause release of a neurotransmitter, possibly acetyl choline, from the efferent synapses of the nerve terminals. This neurotransmitter acts on chief cells, still further reducing the rate of dopamine secretion. This in turn brings about even greater depolarization of the nerve terminal instigating an even greater increase in discharge frequency. Carlsson (1975) has suggested that the depletion of catecholamines referred to above is due to the fact that the amines are prevented by reserpine from gaining access to the vesicles and so accumulate in the cell cytoplasm where they are deaminated.

The forgotten organ of morbid anatomy

As the carotid body and sinus are so intimately concerned with the functions of chemoreception and baroreception it might be anticipated that the morbid anatomist would pay attention to this segment of the systemic circulation at necropsy, particularly if he has a special interest in cardiopulmonary disease. In fact the carotid body is the forgotten organ of morbid anatomy. Pathologists have paid little attention to this organ, confining their interest to its tumour, the chemodectoma, one suspects because it has such a characteristic histological appearance (Chapter 10).

This has led to a peculiar imbalance of our knowledge of the carotid body. Physiologists have been carrying out elegant and sophisticated experiments on laboratory animals for many years, although this has not enabled them to determine precisely the transducer in the carotid body which detects the abnormality of partial pressure of oxygen in the plasma converting it into chemical changes in the cytoplasm of the chief cells and thus into a nerve impulse. In the face of all this activity the morbid anatomist has shown little or no interest in the pathology of chemoreceptor tissue. It is exceptional for him to include examination of the carotid bodies at necropsy even in cases of heart or lung disease where it might be expected to show an abnormality. The response of the carotid bodies in generalized disease is not mentioned in undergraduate texts of pathology. This imbalance in our knowledge has led to the unfortunate situation where most of what we know about the histological appearances of the carotid body in health and disease is based on an animal model. This is very unsatisfactory for it cannot be relied on that the animal carotid body will react in the same way to disease as the human. Indeed the carotid body of the rat, which is used more frequently than any other animal species in experimental studies in this field, does not react to the hypoxic stimulus like that of man. For this reason in this book we shall largely confine ourselves to the structure of the human carotid body, making reference to animal tissues only when this is essential.

One can only speculate why the morbid anatomist so studiously avoids the carotid body at necropsy. In part the answer lies in tradition for, if he has not been trained to include this in his dissection, it is most unlikely that he will introduce such an innovation himself. One suspects too that he may think that examination of the carotid body requires time-consuming preparation and examination of serial sections, which will yield information long after the performance of the necropsy. This is a mistaken view. The carotid body is susceptible to a simple dissection at necropsy and immediate evaluation like the other viscera. We shall accordingly start our account of the pathology of the human carotid body and sinus by a description of its examination at necropsy.

Examination of the carotid body at necropsy

We have found the following dissection procedure satisfactory for inclusion in a routine necropsy and we find that it may be completed within 15 minutes. Following a V-shaped incision in the neck, the skin is reflected upwards to the lower margin of the mandible. The sternomastoid, stylohyoid and digastric muscles are excised to expose the carotid sheath. Following dissection of the jugular vein, the carotid sheath is freed from the vagus nerve and underlying fascia. The common carotid artery is transected 5 cm below its bifurcation and the internal and external carotid arteries at least 3 cm above the bifurcation. Both carotid bifurcations are then removed and pinned to cork sheets to dissect out the carotid bodies. This is achieved by carefully stripping off the adventitial fat and connective tissue with fine dissecting scissors, starting with the common carotid artery and working distally (Fig. 1.3). The tissue is found to strip off readily,

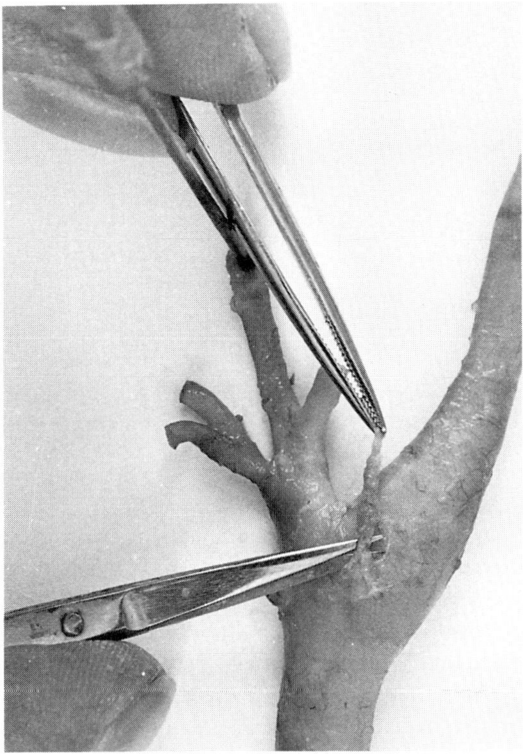

Fig. 1.3 Final stage of dissection of the carotid body. The surrounding fibrous and adipose tissue is held gently with forceps whilst it is cut away with fine scissors from the carotid body. Any remaining connective tissue and fat is then trimmed from the carotid body itself.

leaving the intact carotid body attached to the surface of its artery of origin by its short glomic artery. Where single carotid bodies are present in the bifurcation, this process takes no longer than 5 minutes, but occasionally where carotid bodies are situated elsewhere or are multiple, a more extensive dissection is required and this will of course take more time. It is our practice to photograph the carotid body *in situ* at this point, before removing it to be weighed and then fixed in 10 per cent formol saline. No matter how carefully the carotid body is dissected out small fragments of fat and connective tissue will remain attached but they do not make an appreciable difference to the weight of the organ. Histological sections will reveal how much extraneous tissue has been left adherent and these can of course be used to make an accurate determination of carotid body volume by the morphometric technique referred to below. However, such morphometry is time-consuming and while ideal for research purposes is not advocated for routine use in the laboratory. This question of the errors inherent in weighing the carotid body is discussed further in the following chapter.

Carotid body volume

The carotid bodies of small children and infants are too small to be dissected out accurately for subsequent weighing. The same thing incidentally is true for the carotid bodies of animals used in research. Under these circumstances the more time-consuming techniques of tissue morphometry have to be employed to determine the volume of the carotid body. One method is to apply Simpson's rule as quoted by Dunnill (1968). By this rule the volume, V, of an organ is given by

$$V = \frac{h}{3}\,[(A_o + A_n) + 4\,(A_1 + A_3 + \ldots A_{n-1})\; + 2\,(A_2 + A_4 + \ldots A_{n-2})],$$

where: n = the number of sections;

$A_o, A_1, A_2 \ldots\ldots\ldots\ldots$	=	The area of successive sections, and
h	=	the interval between each section, an appropriate interval being 50 μm.

If a modern image analyser is not available in the laboratory, the histological sections can still be used to determine carotid body volume by the following more homely means. The areas A_o, A_1, A_2 and so on are obtained by projecting each section on a sheet of graph paper with a projector with a microscope head. The outline of each image is traced on the graph paper and the area enclosed by the trace is cut out with scissors. In each instance the area is calculated from the weight of the area of graph paper that had been occupied by the projected image. Calibration is carried out by weighing the area of graph paper occupied by an image of a 1-mm square projected at the same magnification. It is not necessary to weigh each area of graph paper separately because the values of the expression $(A_o + A_n)$, $(A_1 + A_3 + \ldots A_{n-1})$ and $(A_2 + A_4 + \ldots A_{n-2})$ can be derived by weighing the relevant sheets together. This technique does not allow for shrinkage of the carotid body tissue during fixation and processing. While this is pertinent in determination of the absolute volume of the carotid body, it is less important when comparisons between groups are made for the degree of shrinkage is likely to be the same in the different groups. The overall linear dimensions of each carotid body may also be measured with a calibrated eyepiece micrometer to estimate length and breadth. The depth may be calculated from the number of sections required to cut the tissue out of the block.

However, there are now available image analysers for use in the pathology laboratory which allow the rapid and efficient determination of such parameters as lengths, perimeters and areas of objects in a histological section. The generation of such quantitative information by micro-processor technology now permits the rapid assessment of carotid body volume.

References

* =Cited by Adams (1958)

Adams, W.E. (1958). *The comparative morphology of the carotid body and carotid sinus.* C.C. Thomas, Springfield.

Biscoe, T.J., Lall, A. & Sampson, S.R. (1970). Electron microscopic and electrophysiological studies on the carotid body following intracranial section of the glossopharyngeal nerve. *Journal of Physiology* **208**, 133.

Blümcke, S., Rode, J. & Niedorf, H.R. (1967). The carotid body after oxygen deficiency. *Zeitschrift für Zellforschung und Mikroskopische Anatomie* **80**, 52.

Carlsson, A. (1975). Monoamine-depleting drugs. *Pharmacology and Therapeutics; Part B General and Systematic Pharmacology* **1**, 393.

Dearnaley, D.P., Fillenz, M. & Woods, R.I. (1968). The identification of dopamine in the rabbit's carotid body. *Proceedings of the Royal Society* **170**, 195.

de Castro, F. (1926). Sur la structure et l'innervation de la glande intercarotidienne (glomus caroticum) de l'homme et des mammifères, et sur un nouveau systeme d'innervation autonome du nerf glossopharyngien. *Trabajas del Laboratorio de Investigaciones Biologicas de la Universidad de Madrid* **24**, 365.

de Castro, F. (1928). Sur la structure et l'innervation du sinus carotidien de l'homme et des mammifères: Nouveaux faits sur l'innervation et la fonction de glomus caroticum. *Trabajas del Laboratorio de Investigaciones Biologicas de la Universidad de Madrid* **25**, 331.

de Kock, L.L. (1951). Histology of the carotid body. *Nature* **167**, 611.

de Kock, L.L. & Dunn, A.E.G. (1966). An electron microscopic study of the carotid body. *Acta Anatomica* **64**, 163.

Drüner, L. (1925). Ueber die anatomischen Unterlagen der Sinus reflexe Herings. *Deutsche medizinische Wochenschrift* **51**, 559.

Dunnill, M.S. (1968). Quantitative methods in histology. In *Recent Advances in Clinical Pathology*. Edited by S.C. Dyke. London.

Eyzaguirre, C. & Koyano, H. (1965). Effects of some pharmacological agents on chemoreceptor discharge. *Journal of Physiology, London* **178**, 410.

Glenner, G.G. & Grimley, P.M. (1974). *Tumors of the extra-adrenal paraganglion system (including chemoreceptors).* Armed Forces Institute of Pathology, Washington.

Grimley, P.M. & Glenner, G.G. (1968). Ultrastructure of the human carotid body. A perspective on the mode of chemoreception. *Circulation* **37**, 648.

Guild, S.R. (1941). A hitherto unrecognised structure, the glomus jugularis, in man. *Anatomical Record* **79**, (Suppl. 2), 28.

*Haller, A.. (1747, 1749). In *Disputationum Anatomicarum Selectorum* Volumes II and IV. A Vandenhoeck, Gottingen.

Heymans, C., Bouckaert, J.J. & Dautrebande, L. (1930). Sinus carotidien et réflexes respiratoires, II. Influences respiratoires réflexes de l'acidose, de l'alcalose, de l'anhydride carbonique, de l'ion hydrogène et de l'anoxémie: Sinus carotidiens et échanges respiratoires dans les poumons et au dela des poumons. *Archives Internationales de Pharmacodynamie et de Therapie* **39**, 400.

Jacoby, M. (1896). Ueber die Entwickelung der Nebendrüsen der Schilddrüse und der Carotiden-drüse. *Anatomischer Anzeiger* **12**, 152.

Kjaergaard, J. (1973). *Anatomy of the carotid glomus and carotid glomus-like bodies (non-chromaffin paraganglia).* F.A.D.L's Forlag, Copenhagen.

Kohn, A. (1900). Ueber den Bau and die Entwicklung der sog. Carotisdrüse. *Archiv für Mikroskopische Anatomie und Entwicklungmechanik* **56**, 81.

Lever, J.D., Lewis, P.R. & Boyd, J.D. (1959). Observations on the fine structure and histochemistry of the carotid body in the cat and rabbit. *Journal of Anatomy* **93**, 478.

Luschka, H. (1862). Ueber die drüsen artige Natur des sogenannten Ganglion intercaroticum. *Archiv für Anatomie, Physiologie, und wissenschaftliche Medicin* **1**, 405.

McDonald, D.M. (1981). Peripheral chemoreceptors. Structure-function relationships of the carotid body. P. 105 in *Regulation of Breathing. Part 1.* Ed: T.F. Hornbein. Marcel Dekker, New York, Basel.

McDonald, D.M. & Mitchell, R.A. (1975). A quantitative analysis of synaptic connections in the rat carotid body. In: *The Peripheral Chemoreceptors* (pp 101–131). Ed: M.J. Purves. Cambridge University Press, New York.

Mayer, A.F.J.C. (1833). Ueber ein neuendecktes Ganglion im Winkel der aussern und innern Carotis, beim Menschem and den Säugethieren (Ganglion intercaroticum.) *Notizen aus dem Gebiete der Natur — und Heikunde (I. von Froriep)* **36**, Column 8–9.

Neubauer, I.E. (1772). *Descriptio anatomica nervorum cardiacorum.* Fleischer, Frankfurt and Leipzig.

Osborne, M.P. & Butler, P.J. (1975). New theory for receptor mechanisms of carotid body chemoreceptors. *Nature* **254**, 701.

Pearse, A.G.E. (1969). The cytochemistry and ultrastructure of polypeptide hormone-producing cells of the APUD series and the embryologic, physiologic, and pathologic implications of the concept. *Journal of Histochemistry and Cytochemistry* **17**, 303.

Steele, R.H. & Hinterberger, J. (1972). Catecholamines and 5-hydroxytryptamine in the carotid body in vascular, respiratory, and other diseases. *Journal of Laboratory and Clinical Medicine* **80**, 63.

Stieda, L. (1881).*Untersuchungen über die Entwickelung der Glandula thymus, Glandula thyreoidea und Glandula carotica* (p. 34). Engelmann, Leipzig.

Watzka, M. (1930/31). Über die Verbindungen inkretorischer und neurogener Organe. *Anatomischer Anzeiger* **71** (suppl.) 1, 185.

Wharton, J., Polak, J.M., Pearse, A.G.E., McGregor, G.P., Bryant, M.G., Bloom, S.R., Emson, P.C., Bisgard, G.E. & Will, J.A. (1980). Enkephalin-, VIP- and substance P-like immunoreactivity in the carotid body. *Nature* **284**, 269.

Zapata, P., Stensaas, L.J. & Eyzaguirre, C. (1976). Axon regeneration following a lesion of the carotid nerve: Electrophysiological and ultrastructural observations. *Brain Research* **113**, 235.

Zapata, P., Stensaas, L.J. & Eyzaguirre, C. (1977). Recovery of chemosensory function of regenerating carotid nerve fibers. In: *Chemoreception in the Carotid Body* (pp 44–50) Eds: H. Acker, S. Fidone, D. Pallot, C. Eyzaguirre, D.W. Lübbers & R.W. Torrance. Springer-Verlag, New York.

2. Size, Weight and Anatomical Variation

Typically the carotid body comprises a round or ovoid structure situated between the arms of the carotid bifurcation and arising from its angle. When all adherent adipose tissue has been removed, the carotid body proves to be reddish-brown or tan in colour. It is attached to its artery of origin by a short stalk, the ligament of Mayer, whose rôle in the discovery of the organ has already been described in Chapter 1. This ligament contains the glomic artery providing the glomus with its blood supply. The carotid body is thus a pedunculated structure, although sometimes its lower pole extends downwards to cover the stalk and create the impression that it is sessile.

Anatomical variation

There is considerable variation in both the location and macroscopic form of the carotid body (Smith *et al.*, 1982). Thus, although 88 per cent of carotid bodies arise from the angle of bifurcation, 5 per cent have their origin in the internal and 5 per cent in the external carotid arteries whilst 2 per cent are found on the ascending pharyngeal artery. Very rarely the origin may be the common carotid artery just proximal to the bifurcation. It is important to keep in mind that the glomus may arise from one of these atypical sites for otherwise one may fail to identify it or even inadvertently damage it during dissection. Furthermore, in the majority of cases these atypical locations are unilateral. It cannot be assumed that because a carotid body arises from the bifurcation on one side of the neck it will necessarily be found in that location on the other.

Carotid bodies may be bilobed (Fig. 2.1), nodular or double (Fig. 2.2). Such variants are common and comprised no less than 6 per cent of the glomera from both sides in a study of 150 cases (Smith *et al.*, 1982). Bilobed forms consist of two distinct apical lobes fusing at the base to share a common origin from a single glomic artery. Although this variant has been described in carotid bodies which were hyperplastic (Heath *et al.*, 1970), it also occurs in normal organs and is to be regarded as an anatomical variation rather than a pathological change. It occurs in approximately 3 per cent of carotid bodies. The double variant occurs with the same frequency. Here, two distinct carotid bodies occur on the same side of the neck with independent blood supplies. Commonly they arise from different regions of the same vessel such as the external carotid artery. Rarely, however, one may be present at the bifurcation and the other some distance away

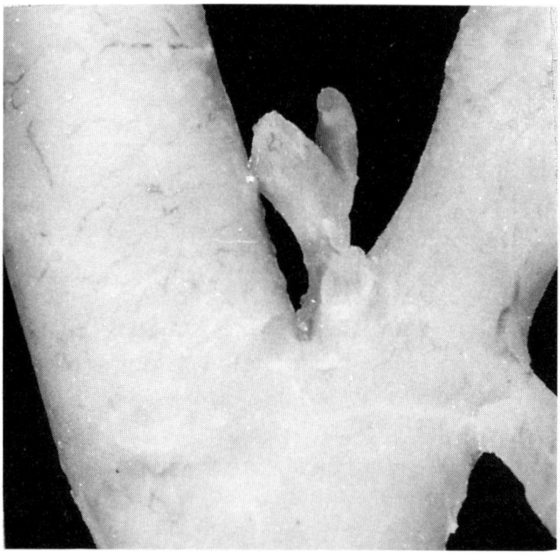

Fig. 2.1 A bilobed carotid body from a man of 65 years who died from carcinoma of the bronchus. There are two distinct lobes which fuse at their base to share a common origin from the bifurcation. (× 4.5)

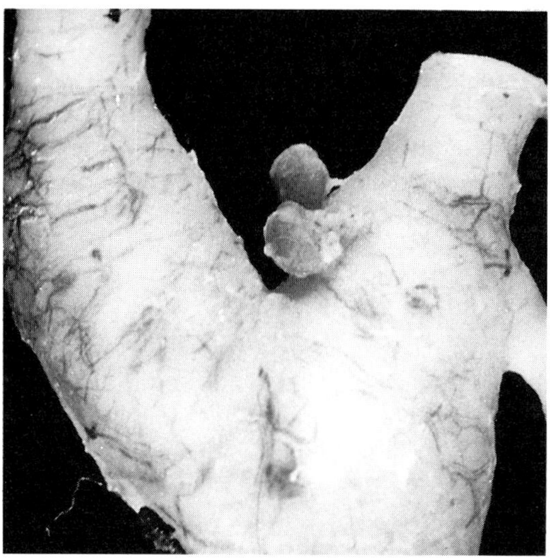

Fig. 2.2 Left carotid bifurcation from a woman of 51 years who died from acute pancreatitis. Two rounded carotid bodies arise from separate regions of the external carotid artery. (× 4.5)

on the external carotid artery. Such accessory glomera could be readily overlooked during dissection. Double carotid bodies are usually unilateral but a single instance where they were bilateral has been recorded (Smith *et al.*, 1982). Both members of the pair are approximately half the normal size.

The nodular form is probably not an anatomical variant but represents hyperplasia. The nodularity ranges from fine irregularities which require a hand lens for detection to large prominences giving the organ a mulberry appearance. It is probably caused by enlargement of the lobules of glomic cells which occurs during hyperplasia.

Size

In a series of 42 unselected cases which included both hyperplastic and normal carotid bodies, the average height, breadth and depth of the carotid bodies were 3.3, 2.2 and 1.7 mm respectively (Heath *et al.*, 1970). Individual hyperplastic organs were considerably larger, the biggest being found in a case of panacinar emphysema and measuring 6.2 × 3.3 × 2.5 mm.

Normal range of weight

The weight of the carotid bodies is of interest to pathologists for its increase is one indication of hyperplasia. It is of course greatly increased when the organ becomes neoplastic but then the change is so pronounced as to make the measurement superfluous. The measurement is simple because, when the carotid bodies have been carefully dissected free from connective tissue, as described in Chapter 1, they can be cut off at their origin and weighed on an electric balance. It is important that every piece of adherent adipose tissue is removed before weighing since in such a small organ this could constitute a significant proportion of its weight. Careless dissection can easily transform a normal carotid body into an apparently hyperplastic one. We have already pointed out in the preceding chapter that the dissection of the carotid body for subsequent weighing is a much less accurate method of determining its precise margins than a morphometric study of serial sections for subsequent assessment of its volume by Simpson's rule. Weighing is, however, much more convenient and speedy for routine use in the laboratory and its inherent small inaccuracies have to be accepted as the price for this.

The mean weight of both carotid bodies combined is about 20 mg, in subjects free from cardiopulmonary disease. There is considerable variation in weight in different subjects. From an unselected group of 42 cases the average weight of the left carotid body was 11.3 mg and that of the right 12.9 mg with a mean combined weight of 24.2 mg (Heath *et al.*, 1970). This series included several examples of hyperplasia and hence these values are slightly higher than normal. In a further study the weights of 13 cases, selected to be free from cardiopulmonary disease, the combined weight ranged from 6.2–34.4 mg with a mean of 21.1 mg. (Edwards *et al.*, 1971).

In a later study of 57 cases with normal carotid bodies the combined mean weight was 18.0 mg with a range of 8.5–31 mg (Smith *et al.*, 1982). From these data the upper limit of normal can be estimated by calculating the limits of probability within which 95 per cent of the population as a whole might be expected to fall. These limits are 6.8–29.2 mg, so that 30 mg may be regarded as the upper limit of normal. Although the mean weights of hyperplastic carotid bodies, as determined by their histological appearance, are considerably in excess of normal, their 95 per cent probabilities overlap the normal range completely. Thus the weight of the carotid bodies is a measurement which can be obtained rapidly but does not always distinguish between normal and hyperplastic organs. As shown in Table 2.1 a combined weight exceeding 30 mg usually denotes hyperplasia but a weight less than this value does not necessarily indicate normality. In order to identify hyperplasia more precisely, histological assessment is necessary.

Table 2.1 The weight of normal and hyperplastic carotid bodies from 98 cases coming to necropsy*

Group	*No. of cases studied*	*Range of 95% probability*		*Mean*
		Lower	*Upper*	
Control	57	7	30	18 mg
Hypoxaemia	5	4	99	52 mg
Systemic hypertension	36	5	54	30 mg

*Data from Smith *et al.*., 1982.

There is no increase in size and weight of the carotid bodies with age in healthy subjects living at sea level. This is in sharp contrast to the progressive increase in weight of these organs with age which occurs in the native Quechua highlanders of the Andes exposed to hypobaric hypoxia throughout their lives (Chapter 7).

References

Edwards, C., Heath, D. & Harris, P. (1971). The carotid body in emphysema and left ventricular hypertrophy. *Journal of Pathology* **104**, 1.

Heath, D., Edwards, C. & Harris, P. (1970). Postmortem size and structure of the human carotid body. Its relation to pulmonary disease and cardiac hypertrophy. *Thorax*, **25**, 129.

Smith, P., Jago, R. & Heath, D. (1982). Anatomical variation and quantitative histology of the normal and enlarged carotid body. *Journal of Pathology* **137**, 287.

3. Normal Histology and Staining Techniques

The normal human carotid body comprises islands of glomic tissue intimately associated with an extensive vascular network and a rich nerve supply in which both axons and ganglion cells are represented. The whole is embedded in a stroma of connective tissue.

Histology of glomic tissue and stroma

At low power the carotid body is seen to consist of lobules composed largely of glomus cells surrounded by bands of acellular connective tissue which extend to the periphery of the organ but do not form a discrete capsule. Instead this fibrous stroma merges with the fibro-fatty connective tissue surrounding the carotid bifurcation. The fibrous septa contain numerous myelinated nerve bundles together with branches of the glomic artery and tributaries of the glomic veins (Chapter 9).

The individual lobules of glomic tissue (Fig. 3.1) are round or oval in cross-

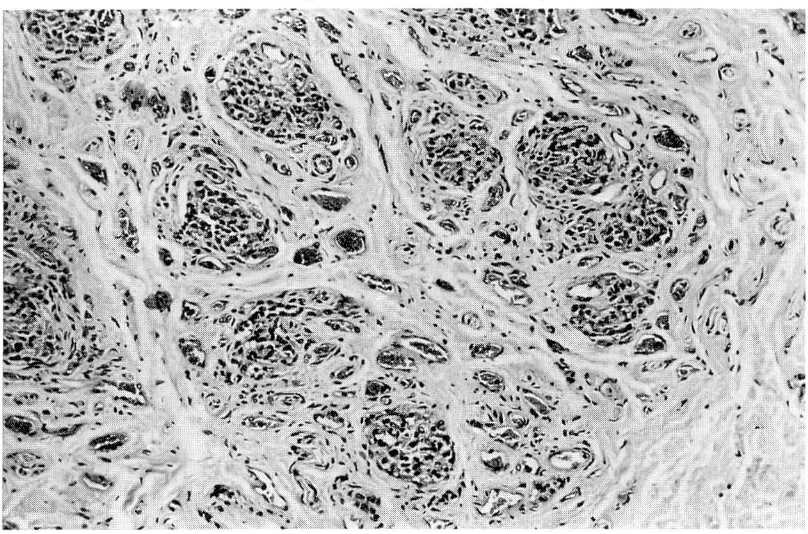

Fig. 3.1 Normal carotid body from a man of 75 years who died from oat-cell carcinoma of bronchus. Numerous small lobules of glomic tissue are separated by broad bands of fibrous tissue in which there are myelinated nerves and blood vessels. (Haematoxylin and eosin × 123)

section but are occasionally elongated and their borders meet the fibrous stroma abruptly. This clearly-defined outline facilitates measurement of their diameter which is a convenient index of hyperplasia when the lobules enlarge. The average normal lobule diameter is about 400 μm although the 95 per cent probability limits range from 250–565 μm, (Table 3.1). The value of 565 μm may thus be taken as the upper limit of normal lobule diameter (Smith *et al.*, 1982).

Table 3.1 Normal values of the carotid body based on measurements of 57 cases*

Parameter	*Mean*	*Range of 95% probability*	
		Lower	*Upper*
Combined weight	18 mg	7	30
Diameter of lobules	411 μm	258	565
Diameter of cell clusters	82 μm	54	110
Sustentacular cell count	39 %	31	47

*Data taken from Smith *et al.*, 1982.

The lobules on closer examination are not homogeneous structures but are arranged in clusters of cells (Fig. 3.2) Each cluster consists of a central core, largely of rounded chief cells, which is surrounded by a thin rim of elongated

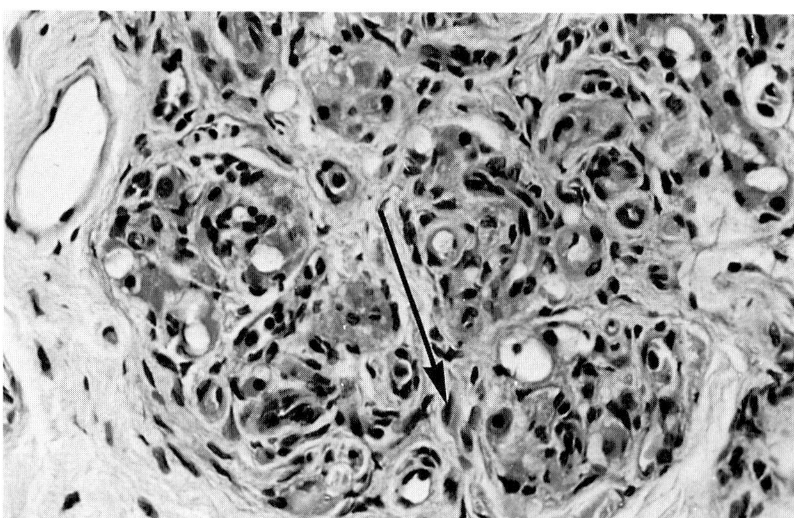

Fig. 3.2 Part of a lobule from a carotid body of a woman of 71 years who died from a subarachnoid haemorrhage. The glomic tissue is arranged into clusters comprising a central core of rounded chief (type I) cells surrounded by a thin rim of elongated sustentacular (type II) cells (*arrow*). (HE × 375)

cells. The clusters are usually circular in cross-section suggesting a spherical shape. At the edges of the lobules, the cluster pattern is lost and the cells are arranged as long cords or diffuse sheets. The elongated cells surrounding one cluster may merge with those from a contiguous one but the diameter of the cluster can be measured if its border is taken as the outermost layer of elongated cells which are arranged concentrically to the central core. On this basis, the average diameter of clusters is 82 μm with a 95 per cent probability ranging from 54–110 μm (Table 3.1). Each cluster is surrounded by a thin, indistinct layer of connective tissue in which there are often small myelinated and unmyelinated nerves, arterioles, capillaries and venules. The arrangement of connective tissue can best be seen using a reticulin stain which produces a typical pattern of fine, black circles outlining each cell cluster and blood vessel (Fig. 3.3).

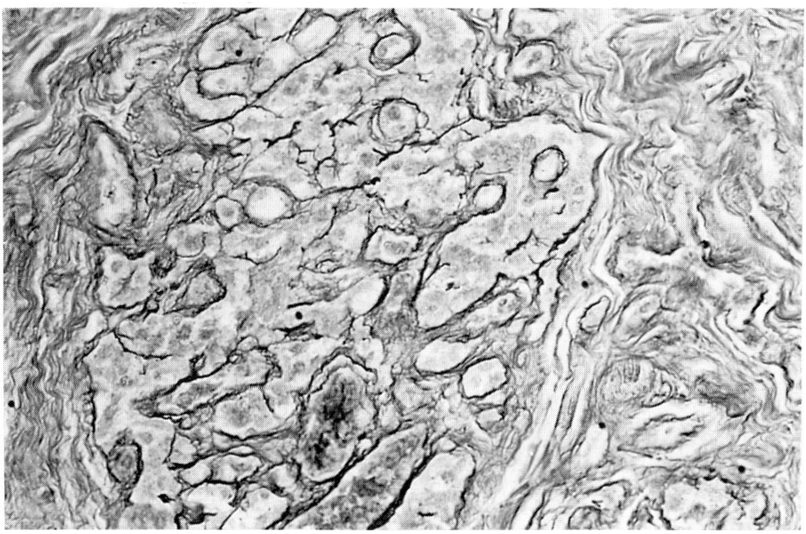

Fig. 3.3 Reticulin pattern in a carotid body of a 31-year-old man with ischaemic heart disease. Part of a lobule is shown in which the individual cell clusters are outlined by reticulin. The walls of blood vessels are also stained and they disrupt the pattern. (Gordon and Sweet's stain × 307)

Nomenclature of glomus cells

In Chapter 1 we gave an account of the derivation of the term 'glomus', which proved to have no precise scientific definition. It will come as no surprise, therefore, to find that the term 'glomus cell' is equally ill-defined. In that chapter we pointed out that the basic histological unit of the parenchymal tissue of a 'glomus' is composed of rounded cells and elongated cells. In this book we shall accordingly regard both types as glomus cells. This is not a universally accepted view and many regard only the rounded cells containing biogenic amines as 'glomus cells'. Such authors believe that the elongated cells act merely in a supporting, accessory rôle (Grimley and Glenner, 1967; McDonald and Mitchell, 1975; Verna, 1979). However, it seems to us that there is as yet no proof that these elongated cells do not play a functional part in the action of the carotid body and their intimate relationship with chief cells leads us to consider them as an integral part of glomic tissue.

The rounded cells were originally referred to as 'epithelioid cells' by de Castro (1951) but this terminology is both confusing and incorrect since epithelioid cells are macrophages in which the phagocytic action has been lost to increased intracellular biochemical activity; clearly such a designation is inappropriate for the cells of the carotid body. Later Ross (1959) called them 'chemoreceptor cells' thus assuming that they, and they alone, subserve the function of chemoreception in the organ. Lever *et al*; (1959) called them 'glomus cells' a term which we do not favour for the reasons given above. The term 'glomus type I cells' was introduced by de Kock (1954). We approve of this terminology and it is in common usage today especially amongst anatomists and physiologists who tend to apply it to research work on animals. The term 'chief cells' is used more frequently for the human carotid body (Grimley and Glenner, 1967) and we shall use it throughout this book.

In his pioneer studies, de Castro referred to a single type of 'glomus cell' but de Kock was able to recognize a second, elongated form which he called the glomus type II cell. The alternative designation of 'sustentacular cells' was proposed by Ross (1959) because they closely resembled the supportive cells of the same name in certain sensory organs such as the organ of Corti, taste buds and olfactory mucosa. In these structures the sustentacular cells support both the receptor and the axons which contact it, in the same manner as they do in the carotid body. They are also referred to as sheath or supporting cells. All these designations are used widely but in this book the term sustentacular cell is used in preference.

Chief cells

In man three distinct forms of chief cell can be recognized, these being the light, dark and 'pyknotic' variants.

Light variant

This is by far the commonest of the three and is so named because of its pale-staining reaction with haematoxylin and eosin (Fig. 3.4). It has abundant vacuolated cytoplasm which is faintly eosinophilic. The vacuoles are extensive and a consistent feature. Many are as large as the nucleus and are irregular and may be artifact due to autolysis which commences soon after death. The borders of light cells are ill-defined so that the appearance of a syncytium is frequently produced. This appearance is spurious and is due to their profuse vacuolation and interdigitation of their borders. The nuclei of light cells are also pale and are larger than the other variants, measuring 7 μm in diameter (Heath *et al.*, 1970

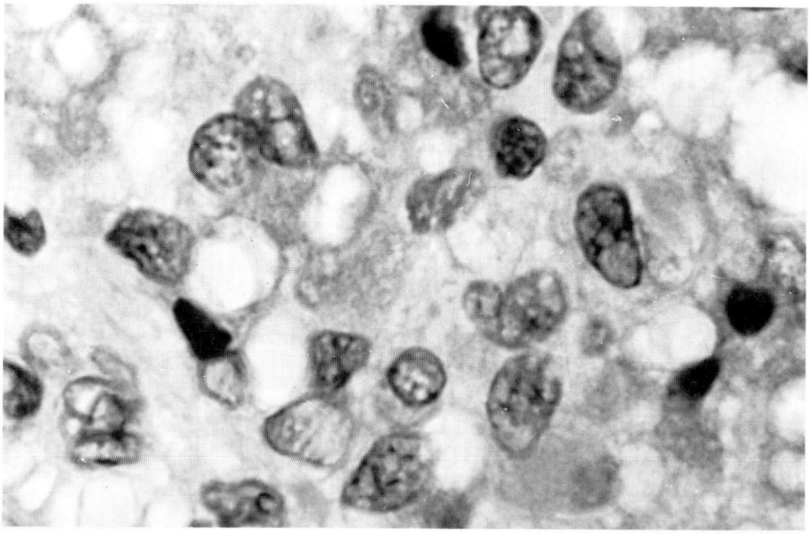

Fig. 3.4 A group of light chief cells from the centre of a cell cluster. Note the pale, vacuolated cytoplasm with ill-defined cell borders. The nuclei are large and pale, often with a stranded arrangement of chromatin conferring a vesicular appearance on many. (HE × 1500)

and 1984). They are round or slightly oval in profile. Their chromatin pattern consists of fine branching strands with large, non-staining areas which are often circular and resemble vacuoles within the nucleus. These strands often radiate from the central, dark nucleolus. Widely-dispersed, small clumps of chromatin may be scattered about the nucleus but are most numerous at its periphery. In a minority of cells the nucleus may lack a vesicular structure but present a finely stippled chromatin pattern instead.

Dark variant

The nuclei of dark cells are slightly smaller measuring approximately 6 μm in diameter. Their chromatin pattern consists of numerous small clumps distributed evenly so that they have a coarsely granular appearance (Fig. 3.5*a*). Pale vesicular areas may be found in the nucleus but they are small and insignificant in contrast to light cells. Overall, the nucleus is considerably more haematoxyphilic hence the designation of dark cell. The cytoplasm is also darker and stains purple with haematoxylin and eosin. It tends to have a more clearly-defined border, although this is largely by virtue of its sharp contrast with the surrounding light cells. Although the cytoplasm usually contains vacuoles, these are small and inconspicuous. Dark cells are heavily outnumbered by light cells but one or two can usually be seen within each cell cluster.

The view that the dark cell is a distinct entity is not accepted by McDonald (1981) who considers staining intensity to be an unreliable way of distinguishing variants of chief cells in the rat. We agree that in the rat there is a smooth

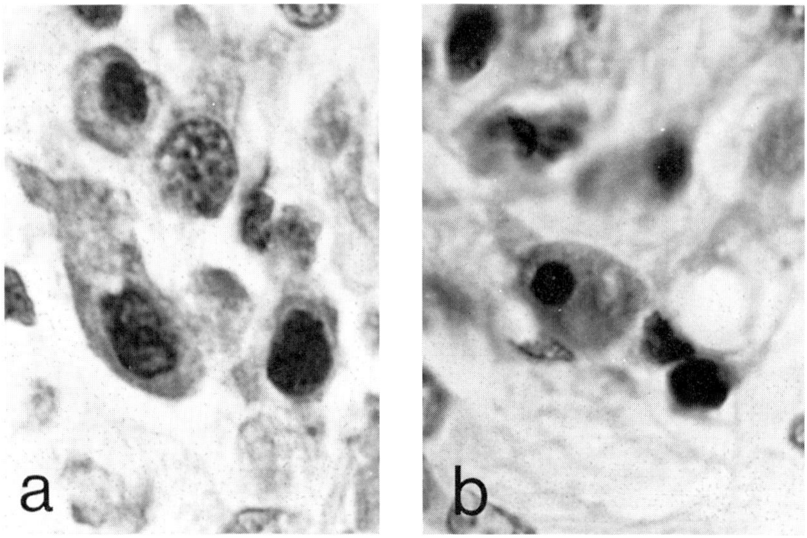

Fig. 3.5 (a) Three dark chief cells with heavily stained, clearly-defined and finely-vacuolated cytoplasm. Their nuclei are slightly smaller than in the light variant with a haematoxyphilic, coarsely granular configuration;
(b) A 'pyknotic' variant also has dark, discrete cytoplasm and a small, intensely haematoxyphilic nucleus. (Both HE × 1500)

transition in the intensity of the staining of the nucleus and cytoplasm over a narrow spectrum from cell to cell but they all appear to be of a single type (Smith *et al.*, 1984). This is in contrast to the situation in man where a sharply defined distinction can be drawn between light and dark variants. This distinction also applies at the ultrastructral level implying functional differences between the two variants (Chapter 4).

'Pyknotic' variant

The name of this variant derives from its small, intensely haematoxyphilic nucleus, resembling the pyknotic nuclei of necrosis (Fig. 3.5*b*). Electron microscopy has shown that these cells are far from effete, neither does their configuration appear to be an artifact due to autolysis. This information as well as their possible relationship to dark and light cells is discussed in detail in Chapter 4. Thus, the word 'pyknotic' is used in a descriptive sense only and is enclosed by commas to stress this usage. The nuclei of 'pyknotic' cells measure 4 μm in diameter, are circular and uniformly haematoxyphilic (Fig. 3.5*b*) Occasionally the faintest suggestion of a chromatin pattern can be discerned. Their cytoplasm is deep purple, like that of dark cells, but is less extensive and rounder in outline.

Sustentacular cells

Sustentacular cells are elongated, or occasionally triangular, and are restricted in the main to the periphery of the cluster. Fine cytoplasmic extensions, invisible on light microscopy, penetrate deep into the core of the cluster composed of chief cells. Their average nuclear dimensions are 13 × 4 μm (Heath *et al.*, 1970), but there is considerable variation in size. The nuclei on staining may show appearances ranging from a pale, fine stippling of chromatin to dense basophilia (Fig. 3.6). Although their cytoplasm is palely eosinophilic, it is

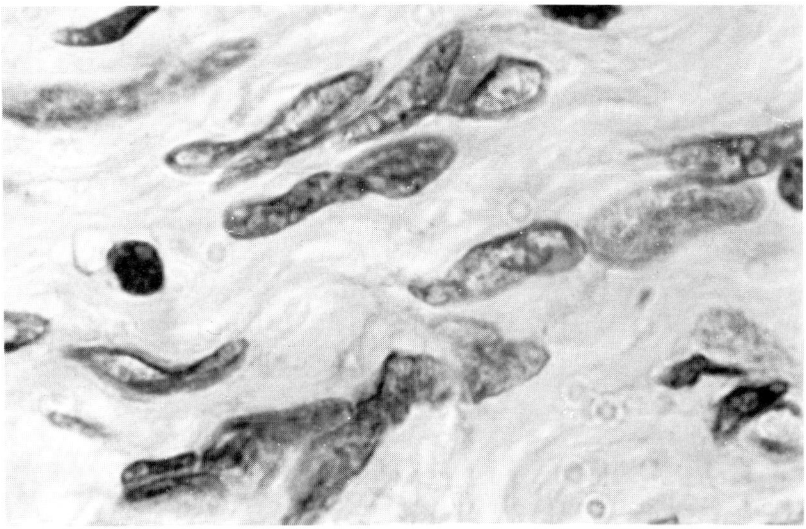

Fig. 3.6 A group of sustentacular cells from the periphery of a cell cluster. Their elongated nuclei show a granular chromatin pattern of varying density. The pale cytoplasm is indistinguishable from the surrounding connective tissue.
(HE × 1500)

difficult to define since it merges with surrounding fibrous tissue. Identification of sustentacular cells is thus based on nuclear characteristics and locations within the lobule.

Sustentacular cells may be confused with other types of elongated cell in the carotid body. Pericytes which enfold capillaries also have elongated nuclei. In this cell, however, the nucleus is smaller, uniformly basophilic and crescentic in shape due to curving around its associated capillary. Fibrocytes are indistinguishable from the darker, more elongated type of sustentacular cells. Indeed at the edge of lobules both types of cell merge imperceptibly in the interlobular septa. In this location the boundary between sustentacular cells and fibrocytes cannot be determined with certainty. Finally, Schwann cells are identical in appearance to sustentacular cells. In the normal carotid body Schwann cells are confined to large myelinated nerves in the stroma and confusion between the two types of cell does not arise. In the hyperplastic organ, however, their differentiation may be rendered much more difficult (Chapter 5).

Ganglion cells and nerves

Ganglia of the autonomic nervous system are situated close to the carotid body but are excluded from all sections in which the carotid body has been dissected free from adherent connective tissue. Neverthless, several ganglion cells, either singly or in small groups, are situated within the connective tissue immediately surrounding the carotid body near its connection with the glossopharyngeal nerve (Pryse-Davies *et al.*, 1964). They are, therefore, more likely to be encountered in incompletely dissected organs. Ganglion cells in the carotid body are identical in appearance to those in autonomic ganglia. Thus they are several times larger than chief cells with large, round, vesicular nuclei. Their copious cytoplasm is finely granulated and basophilic. They are believed to be responsible for innervating the blood vessels of the carotid body and hence regulate vascular tone (McDonald and Mitchell, 1975).

Large bundles of myelinated nerves are prominent within the connective tissue surrounding the carotid body or within the interlobular septa. The small, unmyelinated nerves which supply the cell clusters are invisible on sections stained with haematoxylin and eosin and require a special silver impregnation technique, as described later in this chapter, to demonstrate them as fine, black lines. At the edge of cell clusters the axons form a plexus of parallel arrays of wavy black lines which tend to undulate in and out of the plane of section so that they appear to be discontinuous. From these peripheral nerves a few single axons weave an irregular course into the centre of the cluster, often from one pole. They terminate on chief cells as a variety of nerve endings such as small boutons, discs, menisci or calyces (Eyzaguirre and Gallego, 1975). A single nerve may branch several times to supply more than one cell cluster, or alternatively a single chief cell may be supplied by more than one nerve ending. Sometimes a lateral branch may arise from a nerve ending to supply an adjacent chief cell. The nature of the nerve axons cannot be inferred by the structure of their endings since a single axon may branch to produce endings of different types (Eyzaguirre and Gallego, 1975).

Quantitative histology

Since the population of glomic cells changes when the carotid body undergoes hyperplasia, it is important to know their proportions in the normal organ. This information can be obtained by performing cell counts in which all components of glomic tissue are counted within a randomly selected high power field. This procedure is facilitated if an eyepiece reticule divided into 40-50 squares is used to sub-sample the area. Three high-power fields will provide a total of 600–1000 cells for each carotid body which is an adequate number for statistical analysis. The individual count for each type of cell is expressed as a percentage of the total to give a differential count. A draw-back of this technique is that it provides only the *relative* proportions of glomic cells without indicating whether or not they have proliferated. An absolute count can be obtained by dividing the individual counts for each type of cell by the area of section sampled. This provides an index of cell density based upon the number of nuclei per unit area. If the total volume of glomic tissue is then calculated by applying Simpson's rule (Chapter 1) the total number of cells in each carotid body can be obtained. Clearly such measurements are time-consuming and tedious for all but the devoted research worker to perform which is why we recommend that the practising pathologist restricts himself to the relatively simple procedure of the differential count. He should be aware, however, that such a measurement does not prove whether or not there is hyperplasia but merely indicates a redistribution of cell types.

Using the differential count on 57 subjects with normal carotid bodies we found that the average count for the light, dark and 'pyknotic' variants of chief cells is 54, 5 and 2 per cent respectively, and 39 per cent for sustentacular cells (Smith *et al.*, 1982). Clearly these values are numerically related such that if one were to increase the others must decrease. However, since the sustentacular cell is most involved in enlargement of the carotid body it is the differential count for this upon which we place emphasis. The upper limit of normal for the sustentacular cell count is 47 per cent as calculated from its 95 per cent probability limits. This value provides a very reliable index of normality in our experience since it is uncommon for a normal organ to exceed this value or for an enlarged one to fall below it. This is shown graphically in Figure 3.7 where the sustentacular cell count is plotted against mean lobule diameter in 57 control cases and 43 cases selected because they have myocardial hypertrophy and are expected to show evidence of hyperplasia. The continuous lines represent the upper 95 per cent probability limits for the controls whereas broken lines coincide with the lower 95 per cent probability for the cases with myocardial hypertrophy. It can be seen that for mean lobule diameter the lower 95 per cent limit of the 'hyperplastic group' overlaps the controls by as much as 268 μm. On the other hand the overlap of 95 per cent probabilities for sustentacular cell count is much smaller and equal to only 4 per cent. Indeed out of 57 control cases only 2 are above 47 per cent and, from the 43 cases expected to show hyperplasia, only 4 are below this value.

Such quantitative data, and that from the preceding chapter allow for the numerical definition of the normal carotid body (See Table 3.1). Thus, we define a normal carotid body as having a combined weight less than 30 mg, a lobule diameter less than 565 μm, cell clusters less than 110 μm in diameter and a sustentacular cell count less than 47 per cent (Smith *et al.*, 1982). The last measurement, although the most reliable, is the most time-consuming to perform, but there are qualitative differences in the histological appearance of the enlarged carotid body which can often be recognized without recourse to measurement (Chapter 5).

Staining methods

Sections stained with haematoxylin and eosin provide limited and inadequate

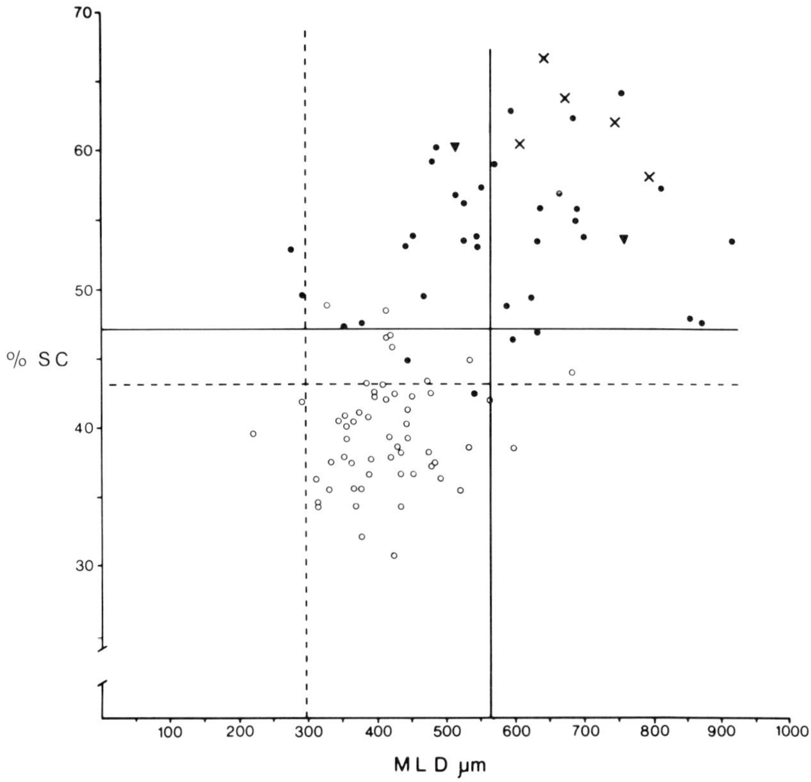

Fig. 3.7 Graph of mean lobule diameter (MLD) plotted against the percentage of sustentacular cells (SC). Continuous lines represent the upper 95 per cent probability limits for the control group. Broken lines indicate the lower 95 per cent probability limits for all the cases with myocardial hypertrophy. Open circles = controls; closed circles = left ventricular hypertrophy complicating systemic hypertension; crosses = right ventricular hypertrophy complicating hypoxaemia; triangles = biventricular hypertrophy with both systemic hypertension and hypoxaemia.

information on the histological and cytological features of the normal and abnormal carotid body. Additional staining techniques are useful and we now consider their nature and purpose. Details of the methods may be obtained from the references to papers and textbooks provided.

Chromaffin reaction

This is of more interest in the rôle it played in the historical controversy as to whether or not the carotid body is a non-chromaffin paraganglion (Chapter 1) than as a practical technique for present-day study of the organ. It relies on the fact that the cytoplasm of chief cells contains catecholamines (Chapter 1) but in the minute amounts in neurosecretory vesicles to be described in Chapter 4. When fresh tissue is fixed in a mixture of chromate and dichromate ions, any biogenic amines it contains stain a golden brown colour. Prior fixation in formalin leads to a negative reaction for all amines except 5-hydroxytryptamine (5-HT) but, if the tissue is fixed in glutaraldehyde first, a strongly positive reaction is obtained for noradrenaline, dopamine and 5-HT and only adrenaline gives a faint reaction. The amines are oxidised by the chromate ions to coloured quinones. Further oxidation and polymerisation may follow. The chromium atoms become reduced from the Cr^{6+} to the Cr^{3+} state and become firmly bound to the site of amine molecules and thus act as a stain not only for light microscopy but also for transmission electron microscopy (Kiernan, 1981).

The technique consists of mixing 100 ml of a 5 per cent solution of potassium dichromate with 7 ml of a 5 per cent solution of potassium chromate (Kiernan, 1981). The tissue blocks are fixed in this mixture for 24 hours and then washed in running water for approximately 8 hours. They are then dehydrated, cleared and embedded in paraffin wax in the usual manner.

This technique gives a strongly positive reaction in the adrenal medulla and adrenergic nerves in which biogenic amines abound. It gives a considerably weaker but still positive reaction in the carotid body of rabbits (Lever *et al.*, 1959). In human carotid bodies there is frequently no stain at all discernible to the naked eye or at best a very pale reaction which is difficult to distinguish from the non-specific background staining of other tissue (Pryse-Davies *et al.*, 1964). Thus macroscopically the human carotid body is 'non-chromaffin', but chromaffin granules can be detected at the ultrastructural level and they represent the 'dense-core vesicles' (Chaper 4) which contain catecholamines. There would seem to be a strong case for accepting the suggestion of Bock and Gorgas (1976) that the term 'chromaffin' should mean the capability to synthesize and store catechol or indolamines. On this basis the carotid body is chromaffin but from a practical standpoint the reaction is too insensitive to label amine-containing cells in it macroscopically or on light microscopy.

Formalin-induced fluorescence

This is a highly sensitive method for demonstrating catechol and indol amines, which works well on the carotid body. The basis of the technique involves the production of highly fluorescent derivatives which can be detected in ultra-violet illumination. Fixation of the tissue in aqueous formaldehyde produces non-fluorescent condensation products of amines. If these are subsequently exposed to hot, dry formaldehyde vapour a second reaction occurs leading to brightly fluorescent products. A brief description of the protocol of this method is given below abstracted from Kiernan (1981).

Tissue, either fresh or fixed in formalin, is rapidly frozen by immersion in isopentane cooled by liquid nitrogen. It is then freeze-dried and, when dehydrated, treated with formaldehyde vapour generated by the action of heat on paraformaldehyde. The specimens and paraformaldehyde are kept in a closed jar incubated at 80°C for one hour. The tissues are then vacuum embedded in paraffin wax and sections cut and mounted without floating on water. They are cleared in xylene or petroleum ether and mounted in DPX. The tissues are examined under a microscope fitted with an ultraviolet lamp using an excitation wavelength of 410 nm. A green fluorescence indicates the presence of noradrenaline and dopamine, whereas a yellow fluorescence demonstrates 5-HT. Adrenaline has a weak, indistinct reaction.

This technique suffers from the disadvantage that it requires freeze-drying apparatus which many pathology laboratories do not possess. In a simpler method devised by Axelsson *et al.* (1973) thick sections are cut on a cryostat and immediately placed in glyoxylic acid solution at 0°C for 12 minutes. The solution comprises 1 g glyoxylic acid in 45 ml of 0.1 M phosphate buffer to which is added 0.25 g magnesium chloride. The pH is adjusted to 4.9–5.0 with sodium hydroxide. The slides are removed from the solution, blotted dry and exposed to glyoxylic acid vapour at 100°C for 3 minutes.

If the carotid body is treated by either of the above methods, the chief cells show a predominantly green fluorescence (Bock and Gorgas, 1976) indicating the presence of catecholamines. There is also a less intense yellow fluorescence in some cells scattered randomly within cells clusters indicating that 5-HT is also present (Hamberger *et al.*, 1966). Although the technique also demonstrates adrenergic nerve terminals, the fluorescence of these fine structures is masked by the background autofluorescence of collagen.

Lead haematoxylin

As we shall see in Chapter 4 the biogenic amines are believed to occur in dense-core vesicles, and more particularly in their clear haloes. The dense cores are believed to be the site of polypeptide hormones. There are crude histochemical methods to demonstrate these regulatory peptides, although far more specific techniques employing immunocytochemistry are now being introduced. Staining by lead haematoxylin was the method originally designed for staining polypeptide hormones in endocrine cells (Solcia *et al.*, 1969). It is believed to react with carboxyl and carboxyamide side chains and is thus similar in its selectivity to the technique of masked metachromasia described below. A 5 per cent solution of lead nitrate is added to an equal volume of saturated aqueous ammonium acetate (Solcia *et al.*, 1969). It is filtered and, for each 100 ml of filtrate, 2 ml of a 40 per cent solution of formaldehyde is added. This stock solution can be kept at room temperature for several weeks. Haematoxylin is added to the lead nitrate solution at the rate of 0.2 g per 10 ml and is then diluted with an equal volume of distilled water. Deparaffinized sections are immersed in this stain for 1–2 hours at a temperature of 45°C. This method stains many, but not all, of the chief cells in the human carotid body a blue-black colour (Capella and Solcia, 1971). Dark variants are particularly well displayed. Although prior fixation in formalin will suffice, glutaraldehyde leads to a more uniform staining. Lead haematoxylin can also be used to stain carotid body tumours although a positive reaction may not occur in every case (Capella and Solcia, 1971).

Masked metachromasia

This technique employs basic dyes which show metachromasia after acid hydrolysis of the tissue. A metachromatic reaction with such dyes as toluidine blue indicates the presence of carboxyl, sulphate and phosphate side chains of polypeptides which have been 'unmasked' by acid hydrolysis (Solcia *et al.*, 1968). Non-metachromatic basic dyes such as alcian blue may also be used. Fixation in glutaraldehyde produces the best results but adequate staining is obtained after formalin fixation. The tissue section is immersed in 1 per cent hydrochloric acid for several hours. The precise duration of hydrolysis varies from tissue to tissue and the optimum time has to be determined by trial and error. The slide is then stained with 0.01 per cent toluidine blue buffered to a pH of 5.0. Chief cells stain a red colour against the non-metachromatic blue background.

Argentaffin and argyrophil reaction

The staining of cells by silver nitrate forms the basis of the classical argentaffin reaction in which substances within the cells, such as biogenic amines, reduce silver ions to metallic silver. In the carotid body this technique is almost totally negative except for a few, isolated, darkly-staining chief cells (Capella and Solcia, 1971). Occasionally, carotid body tumours may show a positive argentaffin reaction (Capella and Solcia, 1971) (Chapter 10). Of more value is argyrophilia, the chemistry of which is much the same as that of argentaffinity except that it requires the addition of an external reducing agent to the section rather than depend on an intrinsic one in the tissues. Silver becomes deposited on phenolic amines and thus the specific granules within the chief cells show a positive argyrophil reaction and stain black. There is often considerable variation in staining intensity between individual cells commensurate with their differing concentrations of dense-core vesicles.

Of the various argyrophil stains available that of Grimelius (1968) produces the best results on the chief cells of the carotid body. It involves incubation of the section at 60°C for 3 hours with a weak solution of silver nitrate at pH 5.6. This is followed by reduction to metallic silver by Bodian's reducing agent at 45°C. Although primary fixation in Bouin's fluid produces the best results, tissue fixed in formalin can also be used especially if it is post-fixed in Bouin's fluid before embedding. Double impregnation with silver may increase the contrast of the silver deposit. The tissue should be counterstained with light green so that cellular outlines can be recognised. This technique also stains nerves and nerve endings but many are obscured by the intense argyrophil reaction of the chief cells. If a selective stain for nerve axons is required, a silver impregnation technique which stains the chief cells less intensely should be employed such as Bodian's method.

Bodian's silver protargol method

This technique was devised as a quick but effective way of demonstrating nerve axons and endings in routine formalin-fixed and paraffin wax-embedded histological sections (Bodian, 1936). Its active constituent is a silver-protein complex called silver albumose or protargol. Sections are immersed in a bath of this solution with copper foil and then the silver is reduced with hydroquinone and sodium sulphite (Bodian's reducer) to give a selective and sharp staining of nerve fibres. This process is followed by toning in gold chloride which improves the contrast of the stained elements. The protargol solution contains a lower concentration of silver ions than silver nitrate which may explain why silver is deposited selectively on nerves. The chemical action of the metallic copper is unclear but it improves the selectivity of staining. As a result, subsequent reduction with hydroquinone produces a rather pale staining of nerve fibres which requires the addition of gold chloride to improve the contrast.

A summary of the staining procedure taken from Bodian's original paper is as follows. Deparaffinized sections are placed in a bath of 1 per cent protargol containing 4–6 g of cleaned metallic copper per 100 ml. They are left for 12–48 hours at 37°C, although longer periods of immersion may improve the staining in some tissues. The sections are then placed in Bodian's reducing solution for 10 minutes. After washing in distilled water the sections are toned for 10 minutes with gold. The toning solution consists of a 1 per cent solution of gold chloride (in the form of sodium tetrachloroaurate) containing 3 drops of glacial acetic acid per 100 ml. The gold deposit is developed in 2 per cent oxalic acid. Residual silver salts are removed with sodium thiosulphate and the sections are then washed, dehydrated and embedded in the usual manner. This technique produces clear staining of the finest axons and nerve endings in the carotid body with only the faintest of background staining of collagen fibres. Furthermore the chief cells are usually only weakly positive and stain brown rather than black. As a result they do not obscure the nerves as with Grimelius' argyrophil method.

Elastic Van Gieson method

This familiar technique distinguishes between collagen, elastin and cellular elements in the tissue. In the carotid body it can be used to outline the lobules of glomic tissue in order to measure their mean diameter. It is also essential if the blood vessels of the carotid body are being investigated (Chapter 9). We recommend either Weigert's resorcin-fuchsin method or Gomori's aldehyde-fuchsin method for elastic fibres counterstained with Van Gieson's reagent to demonstrate collagen (Pearse, 1968).

Reticulin stain

This method defines fine filaments of mature or immature collagen embedded within mucopolysaccharide ground substance. More specifically it identifies adjacent hydroxyl groups in hexose sugars by oxidizing them to aldehydes by the action of potassium permanganate. These aldehydes then reduce silver diamine ions to metallic silver (Kiernan, 1981). Subsequent exposure to formaldehyde may reduce more silver onto the small nuclei of silver particles already deposited. Of the several variations of the technique available, that of Gordon and Sweet is recommended for the carotid body (Kiernan, 1981). This method is not used frequently on the normal carotid body since, although it outlines the cell clusters, it also stains the basal laminae of the numerous vascular channels which rather confuses the histological picture. Its main advantage is for staining neoplasms of the carotid body where the outlines of the 'zellballen' are clearly displayed (Chapter 10).

Stains for mast cells

Mast cells are numerous in the carotid body especially around blood vessels and in the interlobular septa. Their identification may be necessary simply to exclude them from glomic cells and nerves although in human tissues fixation in formalin largely dissolves the contents of their granules. Several basic dyes such as toluidine blue or metachromatic blue will react with the sulphate-rich heparin in mast cells (Pearse, 1968). Aluminium sulphate usually improves the result.

Methods for lipofuscin

Deposits of lipofuscin in glomic tissue are rarely sufficiently extensive to make them visible on light microscopy but they are frequently encountered under the electron microscope. They are more prominent in elderly subjects as with lipofuscin droplets in other tissues. On the other hand chemodectomas may contain much lipofuscin which can cross-react with some of the other selective stains for the carotid body such as masked metachromasia with toluidine blue, lead haematoxylin and the argyrophil reaction (Capella and Solcia, 1971). If such cross-reaction is suspected, lipofuscin can be stained selectively by the modified, long Ziehl Neelsen's method, sulphuric nile blue, Sudan black B, luxol fast blue, or periodic acid Schiff's reagent.

Immunocytochemistry

The new and rapidly expanding science of immunocytochemistry has been applied to the carotid body, although at the present it is probably of more value as a research tool than in diagnosis of disease. Antibodies to enkephalins and dopamine β-hydroxylase are bound to the chief cells and can be demonstrated by immunoperoxidase staining (Polak and Bloom 1983). Using the immunogold technique for electron microscopy these two substances have been shown to share the same secretory granule (Polak and Bloom, 1983).

References

Axelsson, S., Björklund, A., Falk, B., Lindvall, O. & Svensson, L.-Å. (1973). Glyoxylic acid condensation. A new fluorescence method for the histochemical demonstration of biogenic amines. *Acta Physiologia Scandinavica* **87**, 57.

Bock, P. & Gorgas, K. (1976). Catecholamines and granule content of carotid body type 1 — cells. In: *Chromaffin, Enterochromaffin and Related Cells*. Eds: R.E. Coupland & T. Fujita. Elsevier Scientific Publishing, Amsterdam.

Bodian, D. (1936). A new method for staining nerve fibres and nerve endings in mounted paraffin sections. *Anatomical Record* **65**, 89.

Capella, C. & Solcia, E. (1971). Optical and electron microscopical study of cytoplasmic granules in human carotid body, carotid body tumours and glomus jugulare tumours. *Virchow's Archives, B, Zellpathologie* **7**, 37.

de Castro, F., (1951). Sur la structure de la synapse dans les chemorecepteurs: leur mécanisme d'excitation et rôle dans la circulation sanguine locale. *Acta Physiologia Scandinavica* **22**, 14.
de Kock, L.L. (1954). The intra-glomerular tissues of the carotid body. *Acta Anatomica* **21**, 101.
Eyzaguirre, C. & Gallego, A. (1975). An examination of de Castro's original slides. In: *The Peripheral Arterial Chemoreceptors*. Ed: M.J. Purves. Cambridge University Press, Oxford.
Grimelius, L. (1968). A silver nitrate stain for cells in human pancreatic islets. *Acta Societatis Medicorum Upsaliensis (Stockholm)* **73**, 243.
Grimley, P.M. & Glenner, G.G. (1967). Histology and ultrastructure of carotid body paragangliomas. Comparison with the normal gland. *Cancer*, **20**, 1473.
Hamberger, B., Ritzen, M. & Wersall, J. (1966). Demonstration of catecholamines and 5-hydroxytryptamine in the human carotid body. *Journal of Pharmacology and Experimental Therapeutics* **152**, 197.
Heath, D., Edwards, C. & Harris, P. (1970). Postmortem size and structure of the human carotid body. *Thorax* **25**, 129.
Heath, D., Smith, P. & Jago, R. (1984). Dark cell proliferation in carotid body hyperplasia. *Journal of Pathology* **142**, 39.
Kiernan, J.A. (1981). *Histological and Histochemical methods. Theory and Practice*. Pergamon Press, Oxford.
Lever, J.D., Lewis, P.R. & Boyd, J.D. (1959). Observations on the fine structure and histochemistry of the carotid body in the cat and rabbit. *Journal of Anatomy* **93**, 478.
McDonald, D.M. (1981). Peripheral chemoreceptors. Structure function relationships of the carotid body. In: *Regulation of Breathing* (p. 105). Ed: T.F. Hornbein. Marcel Dekker Inc., New York, Basel.
McDonald, D.M. & Mitchell, R.A. (1975). The innervation of glomus cells, ganglion cells and blood vessels in the rat carotid body: a quantitative ultrastructural analysis *Journal of Neurocytology* **4**, 177.
Pearse, A.G.E. (1968). *Histochemistry, Theoretical and Applied, 3rd ed.*, Churchill Livingstone, London.
Polak, J.M. & Bloom, S.R. (1983). Immunocytochemistry of regulatory peptides. In: *Immunocytochemistry*, Eds: J.M. Polak and S. Van Noorden. Wright, P.S.G., Bristol.
Pryse-Davies, J., Dawson, I.M.P. & Westbury, G. (1964). Some morphologic, histochemical and chemical observations on chemodectomas and the normal carotid body, including a study of the chromaffin reaction and possible ganglion cell elements. *Cancer* **17**, 185.
Ross, L.L. (1959). Electron microscopic observations of the carotid body of the cat *Journal of Biophysical, Biochemical Cytology* **6**, 253.
Smith, P., Jago, R. & Heath, D. (1982). Anatomical variation and quantitative histology of the normal and enlarged carotid body. *Journal of Pathology* **137**, 287.
Smith, P., Jago, R. & Heath, D. (1984). Glomic cells and blood vessels in the hyperplastic carotid bodies of spontaneously hypertensive rats. *Cardiovascular Research* **18**, 471.
Solcia, E., Capella, C. & Vassallo, G. (1969). Lead-haematoxylin as a stain for endocrine cells. Significance of stain and comparison with other selective methods. *Histochemie* **20**, 116.
Solcia, E., Vassallo, G., & Capella, C. (1968). Selective staining of endocrine cells by basic dyes after acid hydrolysis. *Stain Technology* **43**, 257.
Verna, A. (1979). Ultrastructure of the carotid body in mammals. *International Review of Cytology* **60**, 271.

4. Normal Ultrastructure

The ultrastructure of the normal human carotid body has been rarely described and our account in this chapter is based on the work of Grimley and Glenner (1968) and our own observations in six cases coming to necropsy (Jago *et al.*, 1984).

Most previous studies have used animal tissue which can be obtained fresh, favouring preservation of ultrastructural detail. Studies in rabbits, cats, rats and mice have been reported by Lever and Boyd (1957), Garner and Duncan (1958), Ross (1959), Lever *et al.*, (1959), Biscoe and Stehbens (1966), Duncan and Yates (1967), McDonald and Mitchell (1975) and Laidler and Kay (1978). The results of these studies are referred to in this chapter only where information on the human carotid body is lacking.

Chief cells

The chief cells are collected into groups at the centre of each cluster. The three histological variants (Chapter 3) are confirmed at the ultrastructural level by their different nuclear and cytoplasmic appearances.

Light chief cells

These are polygonal (Figs 4.1 and 4.2) and have an average diameter of 15 μm. Their nucleus is round or slightly oval and has pale nucleoplasm. The small quantity of heterochromatin present is clumped around the periphery, the interior of the nucleus containing only a few small aggregates amidst an almost transparent background. A small but prominent nucleolus is often seen. The cytoplasm of light cells is very pale and contains the organelle most typical of all chief cells, the osmiophilic granule or dense-core vesicle. This consists of a central electron-dense core surrounded by a narrow, clear zone or 'halo' and is encapsulated by a single limiting membrane (Fig. 4.3). It closely resembles the granules in the adrenal medulla or neurosecretory cells of the autonomic nervous system and, as outlined previously, contains biogenic amines (Chapter 1). The dense-core vesicles also resemble the granules in certain polypeptide-secreting cells of the so-called APUD system (Pearse, 1969). The most likely nature of the granules is a central proteinaceous core, which may be the site of origin of a hypothetical hormone 'glomin' of unknown function, surrounded by a clear rim of catecholamines. Their precise rôle in the chemoreceptor response is

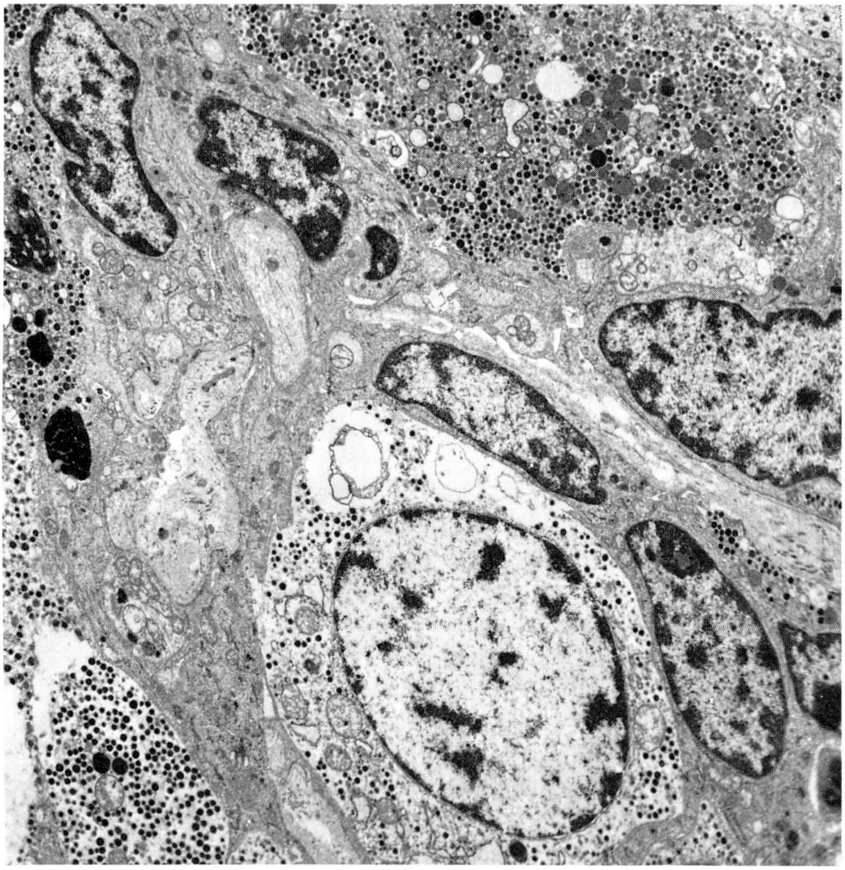

Fig. 4.1 Normal carotid body from a woman of 80 years who died from a ruptured myocardial infarct. The junction between two adjacent cell clusters is shown with chief cells (*top and bottom of the figure*) separated by a row of elongated sustentacular cells. The latter contain few organelles and make close contact with the chief cells. (Electron micrograph × 4900)

speculative. It is worthy of note that dense-core vesicles are larger and more numerous in man than in most animal species. Thus in the cat their diameter has been said to range from 60–80 nm (Ross, 1959) or from 50–150 nm (Lever *et al.*, 1959) whereas in man they range from 100–200 nm (Grimley and Glenner, 1967). In human carotid bodies they are commonly crowded to one side of the cell and show considerable variation in the staining intensity of the central core (Fig. 4.3).

The cytoplasm of light cells contains numerous vacuoles which range in size from a diameter little more than that of a dense-core vesicle to that of the nucleus. In tissues obtained post-mortem it is likely that they are an artifact induced by autolysis. Other cytoplasmic organelles include numerous round mitochondria about 1 μm in diameter, isolated membranes of rough

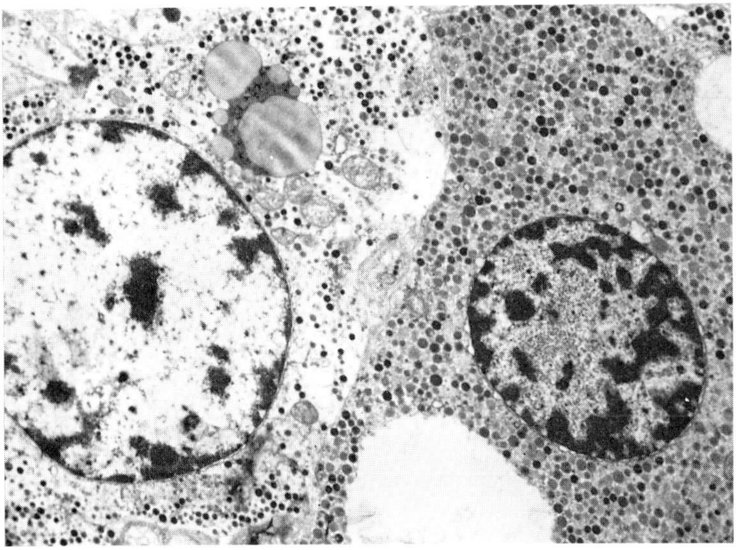

Fig. 4.2 Two chief cells from the same case as in the preceding figure. A light variant (*left*) has a large, euchromatic nucleus and pale cytoplasm. The cell contains sparse, dense-core vesicles, appearing as black dots, and a large irregular lipofuscin granule. A dark variant (*right*) has a smaller, more heterochromatic nucleus and denser cytoplasm. It contains numerous dense-core vesicles. (EM × 5800)

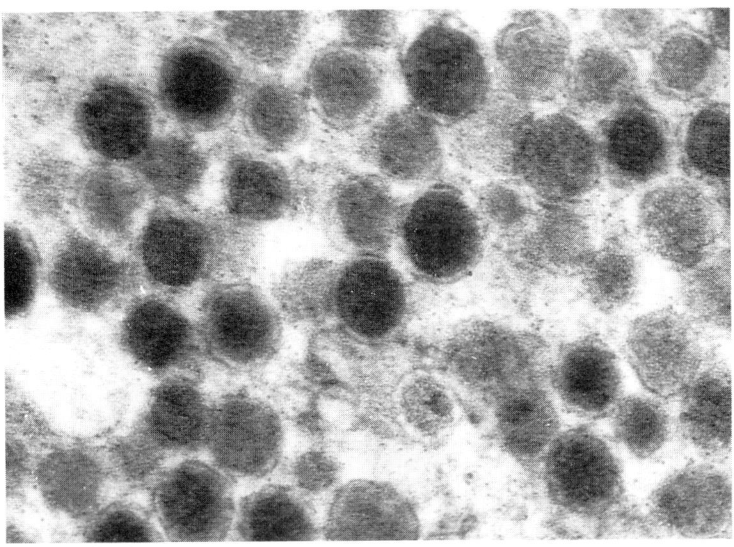

Fig. 4.3 Detail of dense-core vesicles from a dark chief cell. Each consists of a central dense core, a narrow, peripheral, clear zone, and a single, limiting membrane. There is some variation between granules in the density of the central cores. (EM × 83 000)

endoplasmic reticulum, free ribosomes and a Golgi apparatus. The last of these organelles may be very prominent and, in fortuitous sections, the matrix of the dense-core vesicles can be seen forming within their membrane stacks (Grimley and Glenner, 1968). Large, dense, irregularly-shaped inclusions associated with paler lipid droplets are sometimes seen within light cells, especially in aged subjects (Fig. 4.2). They are granules of lipofuscin pigment such as one sees in a variety of cells in the body as a consequence of ageing.

The dark variant of chief cells

This contrasts sharply with the light variant (Fig. 4.2) in that it has a denser cytoplasmic matrix enhanced by the more numerous dense-core vesicles. Many dark cells appear to be packed with vesicles to the exclusion of other organelles (Fig. 4.2). They have correspondingly fewer mitochondria and less extensive rough endoplasmic reticulum and Golgi apparatus than light cells. The nuclei of dark cells are slightly smaller than those of light cells and have condensed chromatin. The heterochromatin forms a broad irregular ring around the periphery of the nucleus and large aggregates scattered throughout its interior. The individual dense-core vesicles are of the same appearance and dimensions as those in light cells so that the chief cells in man cannot be subdivided into two types based solely on the diameters of their granules as in the rat (McDonald and Mitchell, 1975).

The 'pyknotic' cell

This cell, which was not referred to by Grimley and Glenner (1968), is the least common of the three and its sole distinguishing feature is its small round nucleus. This nucleus consists almost entirely of highly condensed chromatin with a particularly dense band some 1–2 μm thick immediately under the nuclear membrane. Two or three large aggregates of heterochromatin are usually present in the interior surrounded by dense nucleoplasm. In some cells the nucleus consists of a uniformly dense mass of heterochromatin. The cytoplasm of these cells is indistinguishable from that of dark cells. Despite the designation 'pyknotic' cell their cytoplasm shows no evidence of degeneration and contains numerous dense-core vesicles and intact mitochondria. This emphasizes the fact that they are not effete chief cells and the term 'pyknotic' is used in a descriptive sense only.

On first inspection by the electron microscope all three variants of chief cell appear to be symmetrically rounded in shape but higher magnifications reveal a complex border. Blunt cytoplasmic extensions interdigitate with one another and, in some instances, prolongations of the cytoplasm may extend for several cell diameters, overlapping with those of their neighbours. Some chief cells are elongated and partially encircle their neighbours (Grimley and Glenner, 1968). The streamers of chief cells contain fewer granules than the rest of the cytoplasm and this makes them appear more transparent. Microfilaments and microtubules are common within these extensions (Grimley and Glenner, 1968).

The recognition of three variants of chief cells is not shared by all workers in the subject. McDonald (1981) considers the staining of the cytoplasm to be an unreliable criterion for this purpose. His objections are based on studies on the rat in which he could produce dark cells by manipulating the carotid body during surgical procedures, or removing it from the animal immediately after fixation by vascular perfusion. He was unable to find dark cells in the carotid bodies of rats which had been left untouched for at least one hour after perfusion. He concluded that dark cells were an artifact, probably due to trauma of the tissue. Other workers have been able to identify light and dark variants of chief cells in a variety of other animal species including dog, cat, horse, rabbit, mouse and seal (Höglund, 1967; Lever and Boyd, 1957; Lever *et al.*, 1959; Morita *et al.*, 1969 and 1970). We think it is most unlikely that the differences in the nucleus and cytoplasm of the chief cell variants which we describe above can be attributed to artifact. While we recognize that variations in electron density of cytoplasmic matrix can be created by different states of hydration, perhaps induced by trauma, we think the striking differences in the number of dense-core vesicles and mitochondria between light and dark cells is a more constant distinction which implies functional differences between the cells.

Interpretation of the relation of dark to light cells is uncertain. It could be postulated that the dark and 'pyknotic' types represent inactive storage cells, since small heterochromatic nuclei are commonly associated with reduced transcription of messenger RNA and hence with little protein synthesis. The paucity of mitochondria and large numbers of granules in the cytoplasm of dark cells is in keeping with this concept. On this basis the 'pyknotic' variant would represent a more extreme form of inactivity. In contrast the large pale nucleus, numerous mitochondria and extensive rough endoplasmic reticulum of the light cell is in keeping with intense synthetic activity and presumably secretion of dense-core vesicles. An alternative view is that in most secretory organs of the body, small cells with dark nuclei are precursors of metabolically active mature forms. On this view dark and pyknotic variants in the carotid body may represent cells which are destined to mature into active light cells. This hypothesis gains more credence when it is considered that some forms of carotid body hyperplasia are associated with focal proliferations of the dark variant of chief cell (Chapter 5).

Sustentacular cells

The sustentacular cell does not contain any characteristic organelles like those of the chief cell. Its main distinguishing feature is the possession of long, fine, cytoplasmic strands which penetrate between, and partially enfold, the chief cells at the centre of the lobules (Fig. 4.4). Each sustentacular cell gives rise to several of these processes which collectively form a protective network around the chief cells. Each process is several times the length of the main cell body and does not branch. Rather it tapers gradually so that its terminations are extremely thin

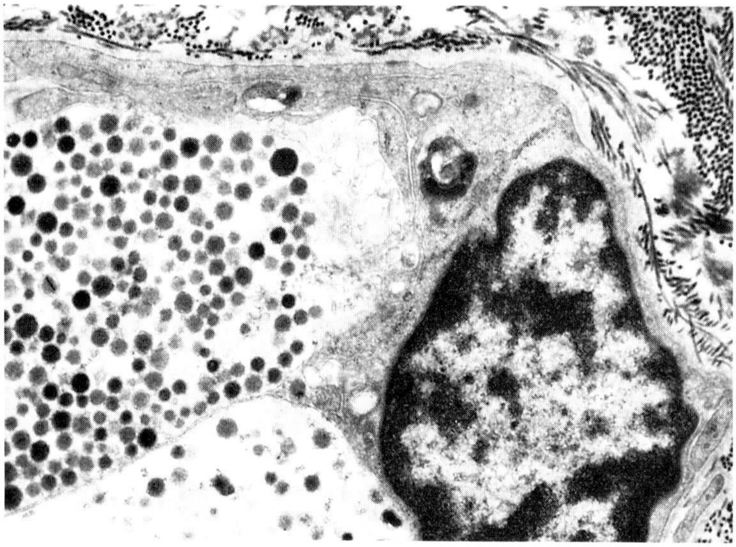

Fig. 4.4 Part of a sustentacular cell from the edge of a cell cluster. The body of the cell contains an oval nucleus but the cytoplasm possess few organelles. Fine cytoplasmic extensions encircle a chief cell which contains characteristic dense-core vesicles. (EM × 14 800)

measuring less than 50 nm (Jago *et al.*, 1984). Where processes from neighbouring cells meet, they simply overlap one another, only occasionally forming distinct cell junctions (Grimley and Glenner, 1968). The cytoplasmic processes also contain nerve axons which they convey into intimate contact with the chief cells.

The bodies of sustentacular cells are confined almost exclusively to the periphery of each cell cluster (Fig. 4.1). Their nuclei are ovoid and measure 3 × 9 μm (Jago *et al.*, 1984) with a wavy outline in places. The chromatin pattern consists of numerous small aggregates within a light grey nucleoplasm, while heterochromatin is condensed at the periphery of the nucleus. The overall staining intensity is darker than that of light chief cells. The cytoplasm contains a paucity of organelles which are concentrated within the cell body. These comprise isolated, short segments of rough endoplasmic reticulum, small areas of smooth endoplasmic reticulum and occasional mitochondria. The cell bodies and processes contain a randomly orientated network of intermediate-type microfilaments but these are not associated with peripheral attachment points as in smooth muscle.

The processes of sustentacular cells usually come between the chief cells and the capillary endothelium. This close proximity to the blood has led to the suggestion that sustentacular cells are involved in the chemoreceptor response. However, their ultrastructural appearances are more in keeping with their proposed supportive rôle, enclosing and guiding the nerve axons to the chief cell in the space between Schwann cells and cell clusters.

Schwann cells

The carotid body is a richly innervated organ and there are numerous Schwann cells associated with its neurons. They are especially numerous in the interlobular septa where they are associated with broad nerve fibres. Here they produce large myelin sheaths enclosing numerous bundles of axons. Nerve fibres are also found between the cell clusters, and some of these may also be myelinated. In this location, however, the majority of nerves are non-myelinated and bear a simple mesaxonal relationship to their supporting Schwann cells. There are usually several axons within each Schwann cell. As the nerves approach the edge of the cell clusters they lose their protection of Schwann cells and are enfolded instead by sustentacular cells as described above. The ultra-structural features of the nucleus and cytoplasm of Schwann cells are identical to those of sustentacular cells. The two types of cell can, therefore, be distinguished only by their location. Thus Schwann cells are normally situated remote from the cell clusters and are associated either with myelin sheaths or numerous non-myelinated nerve axons in their cytoplasm. They do not penetrate into the clusters of glomic cells. On the other hand sustentacular cells give rise to processes which enfold both axons and chief cells within the cell clusters. It is likely that, in view of their similarities in structure and function, sustentacular and Schwann cells are analogous (Ross, 1959).

Axons and nerve endings

Nerve axons rapidly develop autolytic change, and it is, therefore, impossible to demonstrate clearly the axoplasmic organelles in human carotid bodies obtained post mortem. However, the carotid bodies obtained by Grimley and Glenner (1968) were removed surgically in the course of therapeutic glomectomy for bronchial asthma and were thus subject to minimal autolytic change. The following description is abstracted from their paper.

The fine nerve bundles which approach and penetrate the cell clusters contain regularly aligned neurotubules 18–20 nm in diameter, together with fine neurofilaments. They are insulated from the chief cells by the cytoplasm of sustentacular cells until the specialized zone of synaptic contact is reached. In this region the axon is often dilated to form a terminal bulb which contains a collection of small mitochondria and synaptic vesicles 30–40 nm in diameter. Some of these vesicles contain a central dense core and are slightly larger than the others (40–60 nm). They thus exhibit all the features of sympathetic efferent nerve endings.

The presence of nerve endings which are apparently presynaptic efferents cannot be reconciled with the generally accepted view that the glossopharyngeal nerve conducts sensory impulses from the carotid body to the brain. The explanation for this apparent contradiction has not been found in man, but the experiments of McDonald and Mitchell (1975) on the carotid body of the rat may be relevant. They examined the ultrastructure of nerve endings in the carotid bodies of normal rats and animals in which selected nerves had been sectioned. They found that cutting the glossopharyngeal nerve peripheral to the petrosal ganglion resulted in degeneration of 95 per cent of nerve endings. Section central to the ganglion did not lead to axonal degeneration demonstrating that the majority of nerve endings are afferent, and hence sensory. Section of the sympathetic trunk demonstrated that the remaining nerve endings are preganglionic sympathetic efferents. All the efferent nerve endings are boutons, whereas the afferent endings comprise a mixture of boutons and calyces. It is thus not possible to determine the nature of a nerve ending purely by its size and shape (McDonald and Mitchell, 1975). However, they can be distinguished by their granules although it might require measurement to demonstrate this. Thus, sympathetic efferents contain numerous, small, densely-packed synaptic vesicles with a mean diameter of 53 nm, together with numerous dense-core vesicles some 95–97 nm in diameter. On the other hand, afferent endings contain fewer, larger synaptic vesicles 61 nm in diameter with approximately half as many vesicles of the dense-core variety (McDonald and Mitchell, 1975). These authors recognize four variants of afferent ending in the rat. Some are presynaptic to glomus cells, others are postsynaptic to the main body of the chief cell, whereas some are postsynaptic to their fine cytoplasmic processes. The fourth type is a reciprocal synapse with impulses travelling in both directions. Synaptic contact also exists between adjacent chief cells and these may be unipolar or reciprocal.

The direction of the synaptic transmission can be determined from high resolution electron micrographs (McDonald and Mitchell, 1975). The two apposed membranes show cytoplasmic densities on their inner surfaces which are asymmetrical. The density on the presynaptic membrane is divided into cone-shaped, dense projections, but on the postsynaptic membrane it forms an amorphous, uniform postsynaptic web. In reciprocal synapses the polarity of these densities becomes reversed on adjacent segments of the nerve ending. In general there is also a greater concentration of synaptic vesicles in the vicinity of the presynaptic site, but this may be difficult to appreciate where the synapse is reciprocal. Dense-core vesicles of chief cells have an uncertain rôle in neural transmission. They tend to be more concentrated in the region of postsynaptic afferent nerve endings or in the presynaptic segment of a reciprocal synapse and in both situations they could act as neuro-transmitters. However, they are greatly outnumbered by much smaller clear synaptic vesicles identical to those in nerve endings. In this respect chief cells are like neurons and it has been suggested that they are in fact interneurons similar to those in the central nervous system (McDonald and Mitchell, 1975). This concept is supported by the presence of synapses between the chief cells themselves.

It is clear from the above account that the arrangement of neuronal pathways within the carotid body of experimental animals is complex involving several types of nerve endings which permit numerous excitation circuits between glomic cells and nerves. McDonald and Mitchell believe that this can best be explained on the grounds that the primary transducer of the hypoxic stimulus is the nerve ending itself, whereas the chief cell is simply an interneuron which modulates this activity. This hypothesis fits many of the physiological data acquired from animal experiments but it remains to be seen whether it also applies to the human carotid body.

Pericytes

These cells are closely associated with the walls of small blood vessels but since they may be confused with sustentacular cells, their ultrastructure will be briefly described here. The nucleus of a pericyte is usually curved to accommodate its position around the capillary or arteriole. It contains a broad rim of chromatin subjacent to the nuclear membrane accounting for roughly one quarter of the width of the nucleus which is contained in the widest part of the cell. The cytoplasm on either side of the nucleus extends as long, thin processes which partially encircle the vessel. These contain scanty mitochondria and free ribosomes with myofilaments of actin and myosin like those in smooth muscle. They also contain dense focal condensations within the cytoplasm and on the inner aspect of the plasma membrane. The density of myofilaments and number of focal condensations is less than in smooth muscle cells. Pericytes are always intimately associated with blood vessels and do not send out processes which contact chief cells.

Capillary endothelium

The endothelium of glomic capillaries is much the same as that in other organs. It is a flattened layer of cytoplasm of unequal thickness being very broad in the region of the nucleus and finely attenuated in other regions. Many of the capillaries in the carotid bodies of animals are fenestrated but in man this feature is less conspicuous (Jago *et al.*, 1984). Endothelial cytoplasm contains scanty mitochondria and numerous micropinocytotic vesicles in its interior and attached to both the internal or external surfaces. Weibel–Palade bodies are rare in all but a few capillaries, these structures being more a feature of endothelium in larger vessels. Beneath the endothelium is a basal lamina and a ring of ground substance containing isolated collagen fibrils between which are embedded the pericytes. The blood within the capillaries may be separated from the chief cells by several layers of cytoplasm and connective tissue.

Interstitial cells

Fibrocytes are present within the connective tissues of the carotid body. They are occasionally encountered between cell clusters, usually within the adventitia of arterioles. They are more numerous at the edge of entire lobules where they are embedded within dense bands of collagen fibrils. Ultrastructurally they consist of highly elongated, rather dark nuclei and scanty cytoplasm which is highly attenuated in the form of long, branching streamers which ramify between the collagen fibres. They contain few organelles except for occasional small mitochondria, fragments of rough endoplasmic reticulum and free ribosomes in the perinuclear region. Although they may superficially resemble sustentacular cells, confusion between the two should not arise. Thus, their nuclei are much narrower than those of sustentacular cells, they are remote from chief cells and they are not associated with axons. Elongated cells resembling fibrocytes are commonly found in the perineurium of nerves. Their cytoplasm is arranged circularly around large bundles of myelinated nerves.

Mast cells are particularly common in the perivascular connective tissue of glomic arteries and can be readily recognized as round cells with an irregular border containing large electron-dense granules.

References

Biscoe, T.J. & Stehbens, W.E. (1966). Ultrastructure of the carotid body. *Journal of Cell Biology* **30**, 563.

Duncan, D. & Yates, R. (1967). Ultrastructure of the carotid body of the cat as revealed by various fixatives and the use of reserpine. *Anatomical Record* **157**, 667.

Garner, C.M. & Duncan, D. (1958). Observations on the fine structure of the carotid body. *Anatomical Record* **130**, 691.

Grimley, P.M. & Glenner, G.G. (1967). Histology and ultrastructure of carotid body paragangliomas. Comparison with the normal gland. *Cancer* **20**, 1473.

Grimley, P.M. & Glenner, G.G. (1968). Ultrastructure of the human carotid body. A perspective on the mode of chemoreception. *Circulation* **37**, 648.

Höglund, R. (1967). An ultrastructural study of the carotid body of horse and dog. *Zeitschrift Zellforschung* **76**, 576.

Jago, R., Smith, P. & Heath, D. (1984). Electron microscopy of carotid body hyperplasia. *Archives of Pathology and Laboratory Medicine* **108**, 717.

Laidler, P. & Kay, J.M. (1978). Ultrastructure of carotid body in rats living at a simulated altitude of 4300 metres. *Journal of Pathology* **124**, 27.

Lever, J.D. & Boyd, J.D. (1957). Osmiophile granules in the glomus cells of the rabbit carotid body. *Nature* (London) **179**, 1082.

Lever, J.D., Lewis, P.R. & Boyd, J.D. (1959). Observations on the fine structure and histochemistry of the carotid body in the cat and rabbit. *Journal of Anatomy* **93**, 478.

McDonald, D.M. (1981). Peripheral Chemoreceptors. Structure function relationships of the carotid body. In: *Regulation of Breathing* (p. 105). Ed: T.F. Hornbein; Marcel Dekker Inc., New York, Basel.

McDonald, D.M. & Mitchell, R.A. (1975). The innervation of glomus cells, ganglion cells and blood vessels in the rat carotid body: a quantitative ultrastructural analysis. *Journal of Neurocytology* **4**, 177.

Morita, E., Chiocchio S.R. & Tramezzani, J.H. (1969). Four types of main cell in the carotid body of the cat. *Journal of Ultrastructure Research* **28**, 399.

Morita, E., Chiocchio, S.R., Tramezzani, J.H. (1970). The carotid body of the Weddell seal (*Leptonychotes weddelli*) *Anatomical Record* **167** 309.

Pearse, A.G.E. (1969). The cytochemistry and ultrastructure of polypeptide hormone-producing cells of the APUD series and the embryologic, physiologic and pathologic implications of the concept. *Journal of Histochemistry and Cytochemistry* **17**, 303.

Ross, L.L. (1959). Electron microscopic observations of the carotid body of the cat. *Journal of Biophysical Biochemistry and Cytology* **6**, 253.

5. Carotid Body Hyperplasia

Hyperplasia of the carotid body may be suspected on naked-eye examination at necropsy and confirmed by microscopy. Such histological examination may be carried out at three levels. A formal demonstration of hyperplasia, suitable only for research projects, requires absolute cell counts (Chapter 3). A less arduous procedure, permitting a quicker examination of more cases, is a differential cell count but, strictly speaking, this suggests rather than proves the existence of hyperplasia. A simple qualitative examination alone will suggest the condition to the experienced eye.

Macroscopic appearances

With practice the size of the normal carotid body is soon appreciated and variation from it detected. One has to be careful to distinguish normal anatomical variation from pathological enlargement. As we have seen in Chapter 2, the normal carotid body may be double or bilobed; such anatomical variants are not related to hyperplasia of the organ. Whenever the organ has increased in size and yet has retained the form of a single ovoid mass, hyperplasia may be suspected. A very suggestive feature is a mulberry-like appearance of the organ, its surface showing numerous small rounded protuberances. The suspected increase in size is easily confirmed by weighing but care must be taken to dissect away adherent flecks of adipose and connective tissue. The volume of the carotid body can be defined more accurately by microscopy and application of Simpson's rule (Chapter 1) but such precise and time-consuming techniques are not suitable for routine work in the laboratory. A combined carotid body weight of more than 30 mg is suggestive but not diagnostic of hyperplasia (Chapter 2) (Table 5.1). The enlarged carotid body seen in hypoxaemic cases of 'cor pulmonale', associated with chronic bronchitis and emphysema, is congested and mauve in colour, in contrast to the tan appearance of the normal organ.

Histopathology

The enlarged carotid body shows a proliferation of elongated cells around the cores of chief cells in the centres of the cell clusters (Heath *et al.*, 1982). (Figs 5.1 and 5.2). These cells have elongated or oval nuclei and appear on light

Table 5.1 A comparison of measurements on 200 carotid bodies between 57 subjects free of right and left ventricular hypertrophy (control) and 43 subjects having either right ventricular hypertrophy secondary to the hypoxaemia of emphysema, or left ventricular hypertrophy secondary to systemic hypertension (hypoxia-hypertension group).

Measurement	*Group*	*Mean*	*Standard deviation*	*Limits for P = 0.05*
Combined carotid body weight (mg)	Control	18.0	5.6	6.8 – 29.2
	Hypoxia-hypertension	32.0	14.4	2.9 – 61.1
Lobule diameter (μm)	Control	411	76	258 – 565
	Hypoxia-hypertension	596	148	297 – 896
Cell cluster diameter (μm)	Control	82	14	54 – 110
	Hypoxia-hypertension	82	13	56 – 109
Percentage of sustentacular cells	Control	39	4	31 – 47
	Hypoxia-hypertension	55	6	43 – 67

microscopy to be largely composed of sustentacular cells with an indeterminate number of Schwann cells; this is confirmed on electron microscopy (Chapter 6). The proliferating sheath cells commonly have nuclei which are larger, plumper and more vesicular than those of normal carotid bodies (Fig. 5.2). In other instances they are less cellular and more elongated and appear to be undergoing a fibrous transition. They tend to be arranged concentrically as a thick rim around the cores of chief cells which often look compressed or atrophied (Figs 5.1 and 5.2). This cellular proliferation leads to enlargement and fusion of the lobules so that they lose their well-defined, separate appearance. The overall histological appearance is one of cellularity and activity, there being multiple clusters around 100 μm in diameter, although some are as diminutive as 55 μm. As a result the lobules of the carotid body, which are normally around 250–500 μm in diameter, increase in size and may attain a diameter of 900 μm. Thus from a study of a hundred pairs of carotid bodies we came to the conclusion that a second criterion for the diagnosis of carotid body hyperplasia was a lobular diameter exceeding 565 μm (Smith *et al.*, 1982) (Table 5.1). This investigation revealed a positive

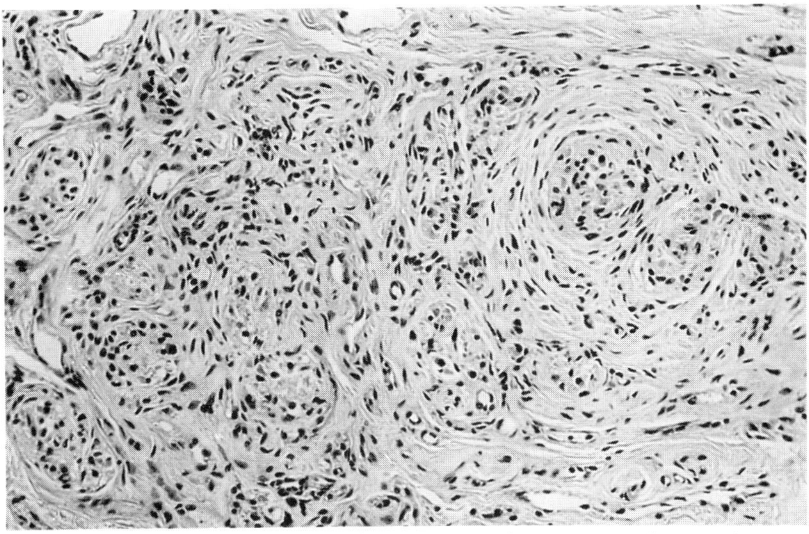

Fig. 5.1 Generalized hyperplasia of carotid body from a case of systemic hypertension. There is enlargement of the lobule. Numerous elongated sustentacular cells form concentric whorls around a central core of chief cells. (HE × 150)

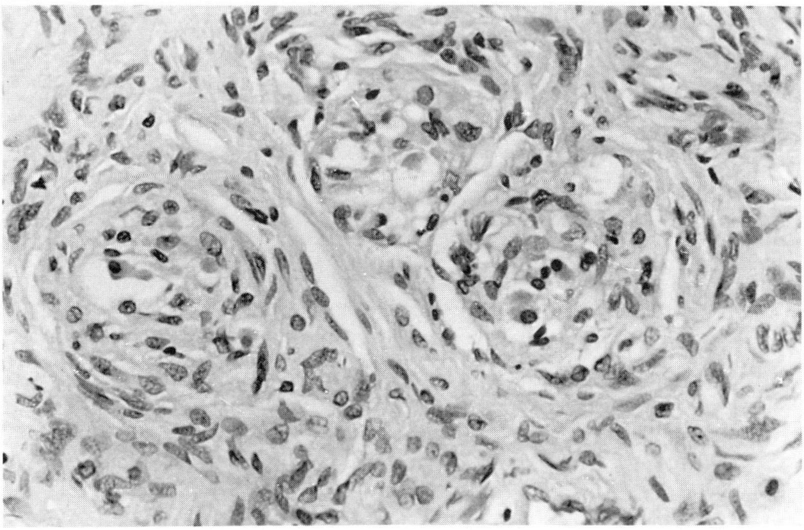

Fig. 5.2 Generalized hyperplasia of carotid body from a man of 72 years with cor pulmonale secondary to panacinar emphysema. The glomic tissue consists of cell clusters comprised in the main of chief cells showing pronounced vacuolation surrounded by a rim of hyperplastic sustentacular cells which show a characteristically elongated form. (HE × 375)

correlation between carotid body weight and lobule diameter. Cases of hypoxaemia secondary to pulmonary emphysema and of systemic hypertension (Chapters 6 and 7) showed a broader scatter of values for lobule diameter which overlapped with the controls. This was reflected by overlapping 95 per cent probability limits (Table 5.1). From our data the upper limit of normal lobule diameter is 565 μm so that a mean value above that figure may be taken to indicate hyperplasia. In contrast we found cell cluster diameter to remain remarkably constant in the control and hypoxia-systemic hypertension groups (Table 5.1). We found no correlation between cell cluster diameter and carotid body weight and hence this parameter is not a useful quantitative guide in the diagnosis of carotid body hyperplasia.

Differential cell counts in cases of carotid body hyperplasia confirm that there is a proliferation of sustentacular cells and in our study (Smith *et al.*, 1982) we found that the upper limit of normal for the percentage of sustentacular cells, as defined by the 95 per cent probability limit, is 47 per cent (Table 5.1). In this study there was an increase in the percentage of sustentacular cells, from a mean of 39 per cent in the controls to 54 per cent in the cases of systemic hypertension and 62 per cent in the cases of hypoxaemia secondary to pulmonary emphysema. There was an associated decline in the percentage of light cells. Usually the mean percentage of both dark cells and pyknotic cells remains low in most cases of carotid body hyperplasia but occasionally these cell types may proliferate as we describe below.

It will be appreciated that strictly speaking the diagnosis of hyperplasia must rest on the determination of absolute cell counts. While this is admirable and appropriate for research projects, it is not a practical proposition for the busy routine laboratory. Under these circumstances we think that carotid body hyperplasia can be diagnosed with confidence by the triad of combined carotid body weight, measurement of lobular diameter and a differential cell count. Using these methods our criteria for carotid body hyperplasia are a combined carotid body weight exceeding 30 mg, a lobular diameter exceeding 565 μm, and a differential cell count showing more than 47 per cent sustentacular cells. The first of these criteria on its own will exclude cases of hyperplasia whereas the third identifies hyperplasia in the great majority of instances. Where the second and third criteria are both satisfied hyperplasia is unequivocal.

Not all the proliferating elongated cells are sustentacular. Some are Schwann cells but it is difficult to determine what proportion they form since the distinction between the two on histological grounds is difficult and indeed some authorities think it impossible (McDonald, 1981). Even at ultrastructural level this distinction may prove very difficult because both cells to some extent ensheathe nerve axons. While electron microscopy will pick out unequivocal sustentacular cells and Schwann cells there is much overlap so that the nature of some cells remains in doubt. Other elongated cells with which sustentacular cells may be confused are pericytes and fibroblasts. Pericytes are similar to smooth muscle cells and characteristically have a somewhat curved shape to fit around small glomic capillaries. They are not involved in the hyperplasia. Fibroblasts are situated beyond the peripheries of the cell clusters in the connective tissue of the interlobular areas and may usually be distinguished by their elongated nuclei.

Increased nerve density

The proliferation of sustentacular and Schwann cells in carotid body hyperplasia is associated with an increased nerve density. Nerve fibres are best demonstrated by Bodian's silver protargol method described in Chapter 3. An increased number of nerve fibres will usually be apparent even on cursory examination but a simple quantitative study will confirm this. Nerve fibres are in the plane of a single section for only a small part of their total length due to their frequent changes of direction, and their numerous branches. This makes it impossible to define what constitutes a single nerve axon and, as a result, an assessment of the quantity of nerve fibre present has to be made by determining the total length of nerve visible in each field. This is achieved using an intercept method as described by Aherne and Dunnill (982). The Merz semicircle grid is useful in this procedure because it copes with any directional bias present in the parameter being measured.

Silver stains reveal a few thick, myelinated nerve fibres running together through the connective tissue lying between the lobules and at the periphery of the carotid body. In the interlobular connective tissue septa towards the centre of the organ the nerves become appreciably thinner and are frequently unmyelinated. These large nerve fibres are not involved in carotid body hyperplasia. Rather it is the fine unmyelinated nerve fibres which tend to follow the same concentric course as the sustentacular cells round the central cores of chief cells in the glomic clusters. These fine nerve axons are regular in their path and branch occasionally. In carotid body hyperplasia the nerve axons are plentiful (Figs 5.3 and 5.4) whereas normally they are sparse. This axonal

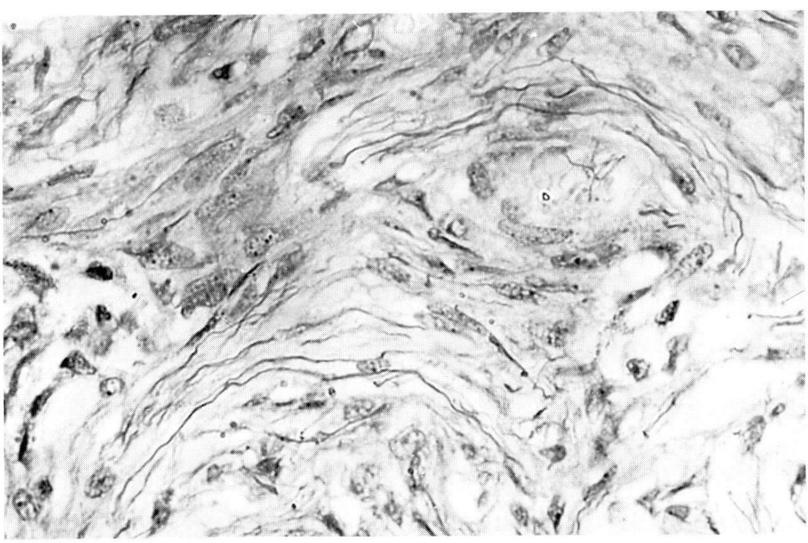

Fig. 5.3 Proliferation of nerve axons in an enlarged carotid body of a man of 72 years with cor pulmonale secondary to panacinar emphysema. This proliferation is associated with hyperplasia of sustentacular cells. (Bodian's stain × 600)

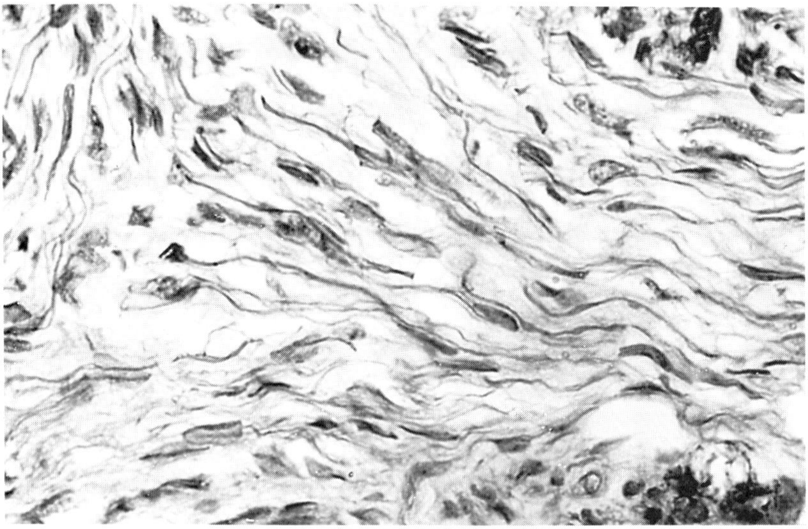

Fig. 5.4 Proliferation of nerve axons in an enlarged carotid body of a woman of 58 years with systemic hypertension. This proliferation is associated with hyperplasia of sustentacular cells. (Bodian's stain × 600)

proliferation occurs whether the enlargement of the carotid body is due to chronic hypoxaemia complicating pulmonary emyphysema (Fig. 5.3) or systemic hypertension (Fig. 5.4) (Fitch *et al.*, 1985). The axons appear crowded together, admixed in the thick rims of sustentacular cells. Large numbers of very fine axons are to be seen ramifying amongst the chief cells. As in the normal carotid body a variety of nerve endings can be seen on chief cells. In the main these are boutons, appearing as swellings at the termination of axons, or calyces, seen as a terminal U-shaped form. Sometimes the ends of axons seem to curve around the chief cell. There are no apparent differences in the proportions of the different types of nerve endings between normal and hyperplastic carotid bodies. We studied quantitatively the density of nerve fibres in five elderly patients who had been free of cardiopulmonary disease and in eight cases of carotid body hyperplasia. Five of these were cases of hypoxic cor pulmonale secondary to panacinar emphysema, one was an example of the Pickwickian syndrome, and there were two cases of systemic hypertension. In the five control cases the mean value of the nerve density was 12.6 mm/mm^2 whereas in the eight cases of carotid body hyperplasia the nerve density was 44.3 mm/mm^2. This was significantly greater ($t = 4.56$, $P < 0.001$). There is a positive correlation between the density of nerve fibres and the percentage of sustentacular cells in each case. Hence in carotid body hyperplasia in man the proliferation of sustentacular and Schwann cells is associated with, and perhaps stimulated by, proliferation of nerve axons.

Focal proliferation of dark and pyknotic cells

In a minority of cases a later, secondary focal proliferation of dark or 'pyknotic' cells takes place on the background of general hyperplasia of sustentacular cells (Figs 5.5 and 5.6). The nodules may range from 40 to 400 μm in diameter and

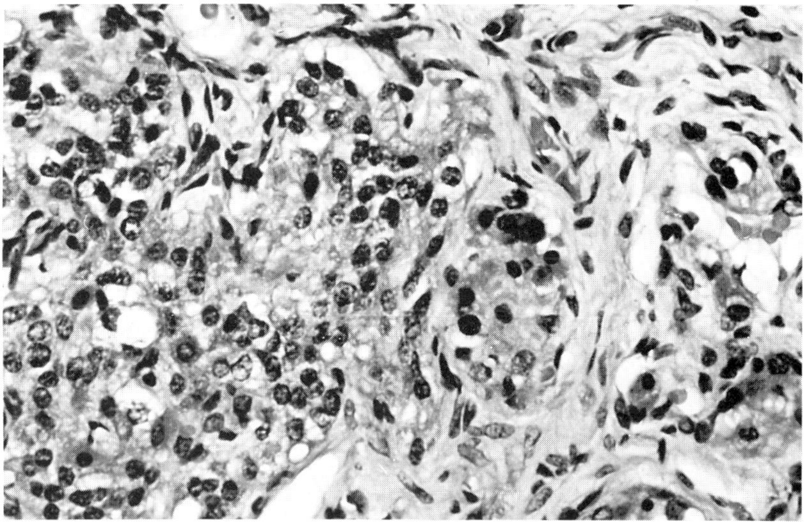

Fig. 5.5 Edge of a large nodule of dark cells extending into background hyperplasia of sustentacular cells in a woman of 80 years with systemic hypertension and enlarged carotid bodies together weighing 33.4 mg. (HE × 430)

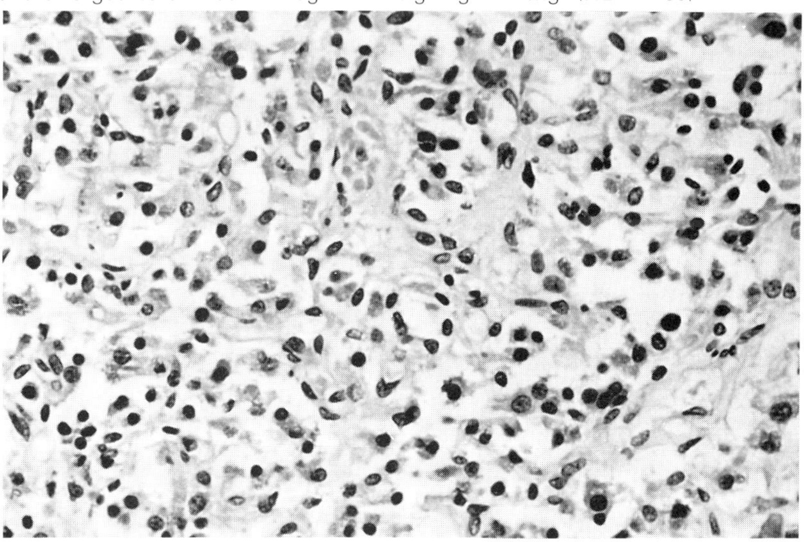

Fig. 5.6 Part of nodule of pyknotic cells in an enlarged carotid body showing generalized hyperplasia in a man of 72 years with cor pulmonale secondary to panacinar emphysema. Together the carotid bodies weighed 60.9 mg. (HE × 430)

some of them may show pleomorphism. In two cases that we reported the nodules were composed of dark cells in a woman of 80 years with systemic hypertension (Fig. 5.5), and of 'pyknotic' cells in a man of 72 years with pan-acinar emphysema complicated by chronic hypoxaemia (Fig. 5.6) (Heath *et al.*, 1984). In the case of systemic hypertension the dark cells accounted for 47 per cent of the cells in the areas of focal proliferation in the carotid body, while in the case of emphysema the dark cells accounted for 20 per cent and the pyknotic cells 42 per cent in the localized nodules.

Nature of carotid body hyperplasia

A consideration of the histopathology of carotid body hyperplasia suggests that two distinct processes may operate. The first is a generalized hyperplasia of sustentacular and Schwann cells to form thick rims around numerous small clusters of chief cells. The second is a focal proliferation of dark and 'pyknotic' variants of chief cells. Since the histological appearances of these two processes are distinct and involve different cell types, it seems likely that they have different functional connotations.

The generalized hyperplasia of sustentacular cells, with an indeterminate contribution from Schwann cells, appears to represent the earlier and commoner process. It occurs both in chronic hypoxaemia complicating pulmonary emphysema (Chapter 7) and in systemic hypertension (Chapter 8). As we have noted above there is an increased nerve density in association with this hyperplasia of sheath cells. It seems likely to us that the proliferation of these supporting cells follows the increase in number of axons. The precise mechanism by which hypoxaemia or a raised intravascular pressure leads to a proliferation of axons is obscure. The demonstration of nerve fibres by silver techniques does not of course identify their origin so the axons shown up could be derived from different nerves. Stimulation of fibres from the glosso-pharyngeal nerve by hypoxaemia seems possible, but the origin of fibres stimulated by hypertension is less obvious.

An alternative explanation is that the sustentacular and Schwann cells are responding not to support proliferating axons but to phagocytose cell debris formed during Wallerian degeneration of them. It is known that within a few hours of axonal injury, nerve endings retract from chief cells and become surrounded by processes of sustentacular cells (McDonald and Mitchell, 1975). This seems far less likely to us for our ultrastructural studies of the sustentacular cells in carotid body hyperplasia have never revealed residual bodies within their cytoplasm.

We have previously considered the possibility that hyperplasia of the sustentacular cells may represent a response to the retention of sodium ions and water which characterizes the various conditions in which such generalized carotid body hyperplasia occurs (Heath *et al.*, 1982) (Chapter 8). Such conditions include hypoxic cor pulmonale in 'blue bloaters', systemic hypertension, and ascent to high altitude with the frequent complications of acute mountain sickness, and pulmonary and cerebral oedema. Should this be the case it seems more likely that such an effect is realized through the agency of the proliferated axons than through a direct secretion, for the sustentacular cells do not have cytoplasmic organelles compatible with such a rôle. Alternatively, the possibility has to be kept in mind that compression of atrophy of the clusters of chief cells, also characteristic of the hyperplastic carotid body, might represent ablation of an endocrine function of these type I glomic cells.

Whatever the reason for the proliferation of sustentacular cells, their physical presence may have effects on the enlarged carotid body. The proliferating cells, largely concentrically-arranged, appear to press on the numerous, small, central cores of chief cells. Such pressure may be involved in causing the diminution of hypoxic drive known to occur in native highlanders and in patients with chronic lung disease associated with hypoxaemia in spite of their enlarged carotid bodies (Lahiri and Milledge, 1965; Severinghaus *et al.*, 1966; Sørensen and Severinghaus, 1968). Such a pressure effect would be enhanced if the sustentacular cells were contractile. Ballard and Jones (1972) and Jones (1975) believed on microscopical and histochemical evidence that the sustentacular cells contain actin-like microfilaments and show myosin ATPase activity This led them to consider that these cells contract, stimulating sensory nerve endings in the clusters of chief cells (Ballard and Jones, 1972; Paintal, 1976). Contraction of thick rims of sheath cells might in excess lead to a diminution in sensitivity of nerve endings. McDonald (1981) thinks such concepts and conclusions premature for virtually all types of cell contain actin-like proteins which form a cytoskeleton controlling their shape and motility.

The proliferated concentric rings and whorls of sustentacular and Schwann cells increase the thickness of tissue separating chief cells from blood in the glomic capillaries but McDonald (1981) does not think that they constitute a diffusion barrier from the blood stream. He notes that the protein tracer horseradish peroxidase (mol. wt 40 000) enters the narrow spaces between glomus cells and nerve endings within 30 seconds of intravascular injection.

The focal proliferation of dark or ‘pyknotic’ cells (Chapter 3) occurs on a background of the generalized hyperplasia of sustentacular and Schwann cells, irrespective of whether this be due to chronic hypoxaemia or systemic hypertension (Heath *et al.*, 1984). The implication is that it is a late phenomenon occurring when the stimulus for hyperplasia has been present for a long time. Chronic stimulation of human and bovine carotid bodies by hypoxia is also associated with an increased prevalence of chemodectoma (Chapter 10). However, there is nothing to suggest that focal dark cell proliferation is a precursor of chemodectoma.

Comparative histopathology of the hypoxaemic carotid body

The form of carotid body hyperplasia described in this chapter appears to be peculiar to man. Although this book is concerned with the pathology of the human carotid body, it is important to see it against the background of the comparative pathology of this organ in other species. It transpires that different groups of species show entirely different histological responses to the same severity of hypoxic stimulus. Thus in such high altitude communities as Cerro de Pasco (4330 m), a mining town in the Peruvian Andes, different animal species will show different histological appearances in their carotid bodies in the face of the same barometric pressure and the same partial pressure of oxygen in the inspired air. We will now briefly consider the microscopical appearances of the carotid bodies of some animal species exposed to chronic hypoxaemia or systemic hypertension.

Llama and alpaca

The carotid bodies of these high altitude camelids are small and show small groups of typical rounded chief cells surrounded by a thin layer of sustentacular cells (Fig. 5.7). The histological picture is quiescent and there is no form of hyperplastic response. Since these species represent the archetype of Darwinian adaptation to high altitude (Heath and Williams, 1981), this histological picture can be regarded as characteristic of *adaptation* to hypoxia.

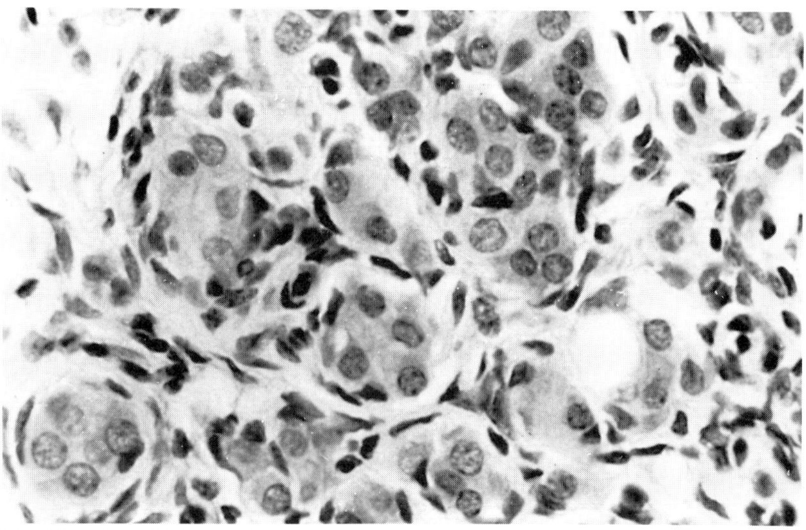

Fig. 5.7 Carotid body of alpaca from La Raya (4200 m) in the Peruvian Andes showing clusters of chief cells, with round prominent nuclei, separated by intervening sustentacular cells with elongated nuclei. (HE × 600)

Cattle

The histological features of the carotid bodies of European cattle taken to precisely the same altitude and thus subjected to the same degree of hypoxia, are totally different. The arrangement of the chief cells in clusters is lost and instead they form sheets. There is an associated focal proliferation of dark cells (Fig. 5.8) (Heath *et al.*, 1985) which is reminiscent of the changes which we have described earlier in this chapter as occurring in cases of pulmonary emphysema

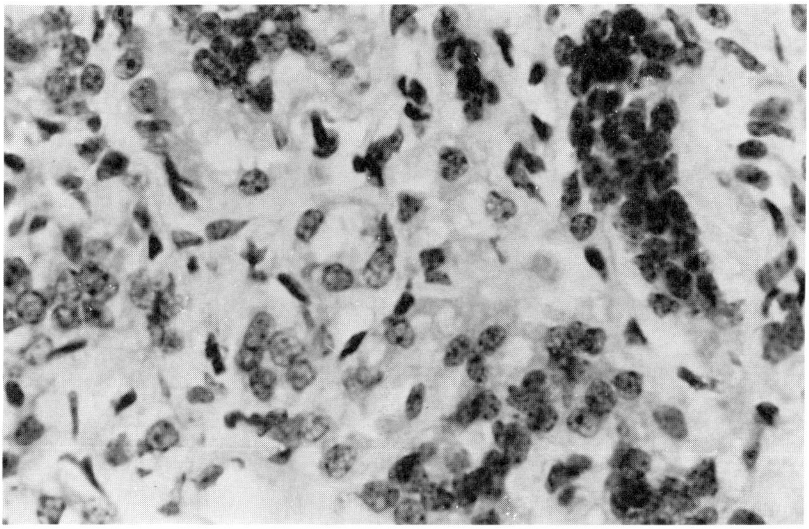

Fig. 5.8 Carotid body of cow from Cerro de Pasco (4330 m) in the Peruvian Andes. Large groups of the dark variants of chief cells are present. There appears to be a transition between them and the light variant of chief cells. (HE × 600)

with severe hypoxaemia. Cattle, like man, are not adapted to hypoxia but have to undergo *acclimatization* and it is tempting to associate the histological features we describe with this biological process. However, it has to be kept in mind that the carotid bodies of cattle at low altitude also show focal collections of dark cells (Heath *et al.*, 1985). The carotid bodies of cattle at high altitude are enlarged and there is an increased prevalence of chemodectoma (Chapter 10).

Guinea pig, rabbit and dog

These species show a distinct type of histological reaction. The carotid bodies are enlarged. Sections show a characteristic pallor with pronounced vacuolation of chief cells (Fig. 5.9). This is based on vacuolation and enlargement of the dense-core vesicles as described in Chapter 6. The clusters of chief cells are increased in size and this leads to an enlargement of the packets surrounded and delineated by reticulin fibrils. In none of these species did we find focal dark cell proliferation or sustentacular cell hyperplasia (Edwards *et al.*, 1971; Heath *et al.*, 1985).

Rat

Wistar albino rats exposed to simulated high altitude in a decompression chamber show an acute, reversible, enlargement of the carotid bodies due largely to vascular engorgement (Heath *et al.*, 1985). Spontaneously hypertensive rats of the Okamoto strain show enlargement due to proliferation of both chief and sustentacular cells so that there is no change in the differential count (Smith *et al.*, 1984).

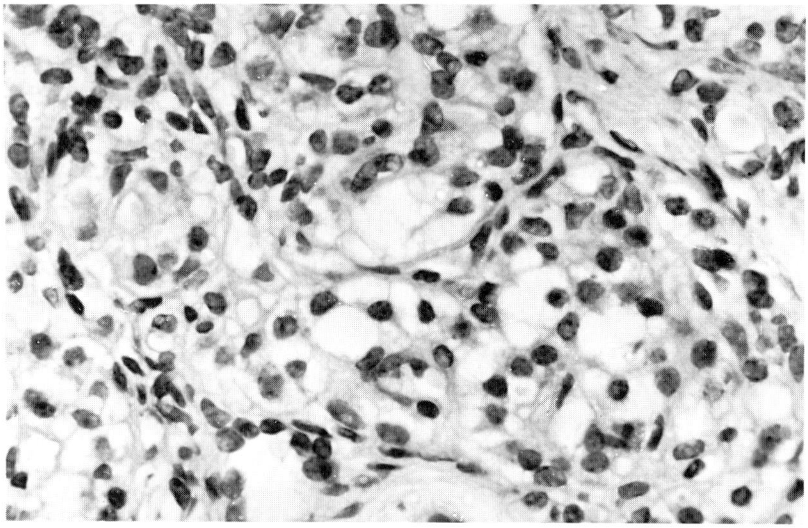

Fig. 5.9 Enlarged carotid body of high-altitude guinea pig from Cerro de Pasco (4330 m) in the Peruvian Andes. The hyperplastic light variants of chief cells show pronounced cytoplasmic vacuolation. (HE × 504)

Conclusion

There is a general awareness that the results of experiments on animals and the interpretation of histological studies of tissue arising from them must be applied to the human situation with great circumspection. The brief descriptions given here have shown that this certainly applies to the histopathology of the carotid body.

References

Aherne, W.A. & Dunnill, M.S. (1982). *Morphometry* (p. 163). Edward Arnold, London.

Ballard, K.J. & Jones, J.V. (1972). Demonstration of choline acetyl transferase activity in the carotid body of the cat. *Journal of Physiology* (Lond.) **227**, 87.

de Castro F. (1926). Sur la structure et l'innervation de la glande intercarotidienne (glomus caroticum) de l'homme et des mammifères, et sur un nouveau systeme d'innervation autonome du nerf glossopharyngien. *Trabajas del laboratorio de investigaciones Biologicas de la Universidad de Madrid* **24**, 365.

Edwards, C., Heath, D., Harris, P., Castillo, Y., Krüger, H. & Arias-Stella, J. (1971). The carotid body in animals at high altitude. *Journal of Pathology* **104**, 231.

Fitch, R., Smith, P. & Heath, D. (1985). A quantitative study of nerve axons in carotid body hyperplasia. *Archives of Pathology*. In Press.

Heath, D., Smith, P. & Jago, R. (1982). Hyperplasia of the carotid body. *Journal of Pathology* **138**, 115.

Heath, D., Smith, P. & Jago, R. (1984). Dark cell proliferation in carotid body hyperplasia. *Journal of Pathology* **142**, 39.

Heath, D., Smith, P., Fitch, R. & Harris, P. (1985). Comparative pathology of the enlarged carotid body. *Journal of Comparative Pathology*. In Press.

Heath, D. & Williams, D.R. (1981). *Man at High Altitude, The Pathophysiology of Acclimatization and Adaptation* (Second edition). Churchill Livingstone, Edinburgh.

Jones, J.V. (1975). Localization and quantitation of the carotid body enzymes: their relevance to the cholinergic transmitter hypothesis. In: *The Peripheral Chemoreceptors* (pp 143-62). Ed: M.J. Purves. New York, Cambridge University Press.

Lahiri, S. & Milledge, J.S. (1965). Sherpa physiology. *Nature, London* **207**, 610.

McDonald, D.M. (1981). Peripheral chemoreceptors. Structure-function relationships of the carotid body. In: *Regulation of Breathing* (p. 105). Ed: T.F. Hornbein. Marcel Dekker, New York.

McDonald, D.M. & Mitchell, R.A. (1975). The innervation of glomus cells, ganglion cells and blood vessels in the rat carotid body: a quantitative ultrastructural analysis. *Journal of Neurocytology* **4**, 177.

Paintal, A.S. (1976). Mechanism transmission of sensory information at chemoreceptors. In: *Morphology and Mechanisms of Chemoreceptors* (pp 121-30). Ed: A.S. Paintal. Vallabhbhai Patel Chest Inst., Delhi.

Severinghaus, J.W., Bainton, C.R. & Carcelan, A. (1966). Respiratory insensitivity to hypoxia in chronically hypoxic man. *Respiration Physiology* , 308.

Smith, P., Jago, R. & Heath, D. (1982). Anatomical variation and quantitative histology of the normal and enlarged carotid body. *Journal of Pathology* **137**, 287.

Smith, P., Jago, R. & Heath, D. (1984). Glomic cells and blood vessels in the hyperplastic carotid bodies of spontaneously hypertensive rats. *Cardiovascular Research* **18**, 471.

Sørensen, S.C. & Severinghaus, J.W. (1968). Irreversible respiratory insensitivity to acute hypoxia in man born at high altitude. *Journal of Applied Physiology* **25**, 217.

6. Ultrastructure of the Hyperplastic and Hypoxic Carotid Body

In this chapter we describe the ultrastructural appearances of generalized hyperplasia and focal proliferation of dark cells in the human carotid body. We also give an account of the changes which occur in the dense-core vesicles of carotid bodies of animals exposed to acute hypoxia and chronic exposure to natural and simulated high altitude.

Generalized hyperplasia

Electron micrographs confirm the same cellular arrangement as seen on light microscopy, the most noteable feature being thick bands of elongated cells around the cores of chief cells (Jago *et al.*, 1984). These proliferating tissues show ultrastructural features consistent with their being composed of sustentacular cells. Thus they have long nuclei and a rather attenuated cytoplasm showing a paucity of organelles except for fascicles of intermediate filaments. At the same time many of these cells are atypical, as they are associated with several axons rather than the expected one or two (Figs 6.1 and 6.2). Furthermore, their nuclei are commonly broader and paler than normal so that, when cut transversely, they are reminiscent of those of the light chief cell.

Precise identification of these elongated cells as sustentacular is commonly difficult for they closely resemble Schwann cells at ultrastructural level. Elongated cells adjacent to the central cores of chief cells send out processes to enfold them and contain numerous nerve axons; they are indisputably sustentacular. Cells of similar configuration which are situated at the periphery of the central core, and commonly associated with nerve bundles and myelin sheaths, are certainly Schwann cells. The problem arises in the designation of elongated cells situated in an intermediate position and commonly showing the broad, pale nuclei referred to above. They are best regarded as a mixture of sustentacular and Schwann cells in unknown proportions and indeed the problem is largely one of semantics. One difficulty in precise identification is the occasional finding of small, immature myelin sheaths within some cells which otherwise fulfil the criteria for being sustentacular cells. There is a prominent increase in the number of axons around each cell cluster and the proliferation of sustentacular and Schwann cells may represent a reponse to this.

Within the central cores of chief cells there is often an increase in the number of cytoplasmic processes from sustentacular cells. This is associated with an

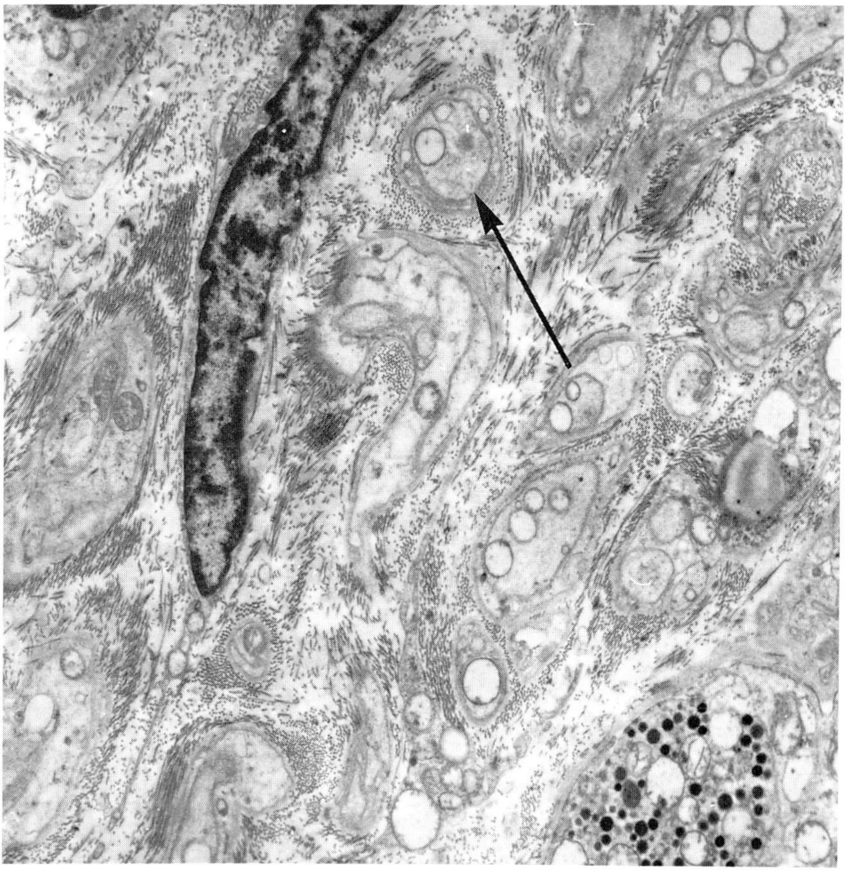

Fig. 6.1 Hyperplastic carotid body from a woman of 80 years with systemic hypertension. Numerous nerve axons (*arrow*) are embedded within the cytoplasm of sustentacular and Schwann cells around the periphery of a cell cluster. The nucleus of one of these elongated cells is seen on the left. (EM × 7000)

apparent increase in the number of axons contacting chief cells, although not as many as one might anticipate from their large numbers at the periphery. The chief cells themselves show no abnormality and in particular their dense-core vesicles are not vacuolated or altered in number. This is in striking contrast to the intense vacuolation which occurs in the chief cells of the enlarged carotid bodies of some animals at high altitude like the guinea pig and rabbit (Chapter 5). The cytoplasmic vacuoles in these species are believed to form from fusion of enlarged, depleted dense-core vesicles as described later in this chapter.

A small minority of the elongated cells are fibroblasts. They have narrower, darker nuclei and are confined largely to the periphery of lobules where they form a thin layer outside the main mass of sustentacular and Schwann cells (Fig. 6.3). Many of them are inactive with scanty, finely attenuated cytoplasm as in the normal carotid body (Chapter 4), but others are broader with extensive,

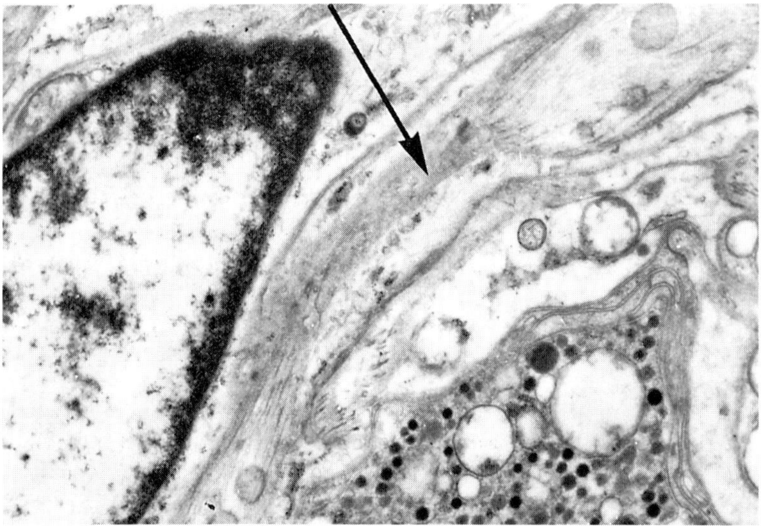

Fig. 6.2 Part of a sustentacular cell, the nucleus of which is seen to the left, makes close contact with a chief cell (*lower right*). A nerve axon containing neurotubules (*arrow*) runs through the cytoplasm of the sustentacular cell. (EM × 12 200)

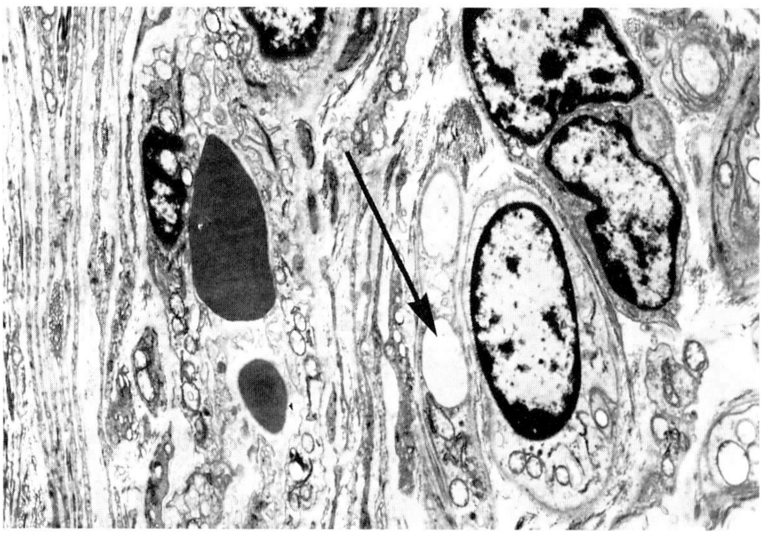

Fig. 6.3 Hyperplastic carotid body from the same case as in Fig. 6.1. A capillary (*centre*) is situated at the edge of a glomic lobule and is surrounded by numerous cytoplasmic prolongations of fibrocytes. Deeper into the lobule (*right*) there are sustentacular and Schwann cells with their associated axons (*arrow*). (EM × 4700)

dilated, rough endoplasmic reticulum and prominent Golgi apparatus typical of active fibroblasts. They are associated with ground substance and collagen fibrils. Whether these fibroblasts originate from activation of pre-existing fibrocytes or from an alteration in the function of Schwann cells is unknown. Suffice it to say that there is an element of fibrosis in carotid body hyperplasia. In contrast, pericytes are not so involved.

Carotid body hyperplasia thus involves both a proliferation of Schwann and sustentacular cells and an increase in the number of axons. The latter process almost certainly does not involve an increase in the number of neurons, but rather an increased arborization of their axonal branches in the region of the glomic lobules. The pronounced proliferation of sustentacular and Schwann cells may represent a passive response to the need for increased axonal support. There is no evidence that the axons are sensory and derived from the glossopharyngeal nerve as they could equally well be sympathetic in origin. As a consequence it is impossible to assess the physiological significance of their proliferation. Reference has already been made to the fact that the enlarged carotid body in states of chronic hypoxia is associated with a diminished hypoxic drive. This may be associated with destruction of chief cells which might stimulate proliferation of nerve axons, perhaps in an attempt to improve chemoreceptor function following impaired sensitivity. This would be comparable to the proliferation of nerve axons in muscle following destruction of muscle cells.

Sustentacular cells share with Schwann cells the capacity to phagocytose cellular debris formed during Wallerian degeneration (McDonald and Mitchell, 1975) and thus they may proliferate in response to degeneration of nerves in the carotid body. While there is yet insufficient evidence to support or refute this notion, it is worthy of note that sustentacular cells do not contain cellular fragments and myelin figures as they would had they ingested necrotic axoplasm, unless the rudimentary myelin sheaths are in reality residual bodies of phagocytosis.

Focal proliferation of dark cells

The ultrastructure of dark cells in focal hyperplastic nodules (Chapter 5) differs in several respects from that of the normal dark variant. There is considerable pleomorphism so that the nucleus assumes a variety of shapes with many infoldings of its membrane in contrast to the rounded form typical of the normal dark cell (Fig. 6.4). There is also unusual variability in the electron density of the nucleoplasm. Within the cytoplasm there are several large, round mitochondria and irregular cisternae of rough endoplasmic reticulum which do not feature in the normal cell. Also characteristic is the wide range in the number of dense-core vesicles, such that some cells contain a relative paucity whereas others are loaded with them. There is an exceptional variation in diameter of the vesicles ranging from 50–600 nm. Many empty microvacuoles are present in the cytoplasm, some being as large as 800 nm and apparently merging with the osmiophilic vesicles. The cytoplasmic outline of dark cells is irregular with many cells having numerous short, branching processes.

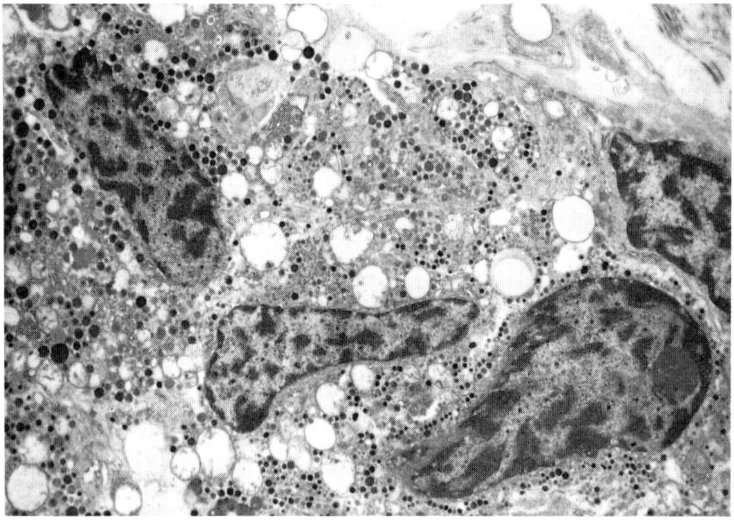

Fig. 6.4 A focal nodule of dark cell hyperplasia found in the same case. Note the irregular shape of the nuclei. The cytoplasm contains numerous dense-core vesicles which have a variable diameter and staining intensity. There are several small vacuoles in the cytoplasm. (EM × 5600)

Effects of acute hypoxia on the ultrastructure of dense-core vesicles

If one accepts that the glomic chief cell is sensitive to hypoxia either as a transducer or a modulator of a neural response, one might expect to see changes in its cytoplasm in states of hypoxaemia. Furthermore, if it is the dense-core vesicle which is the effector part of the cell, alterations in the structure or distribution of this organelle should be visible. Such changes have been described only in animals but even in them the experimental evidence is often contradictory. In one of the first experiments on the effect of acute hypoxia on dense-core vesicles, rats were subjected to severe hypoxia by exposing them to air in which the oxygen concentration was only 2.5 per cent for periods ranging from 5–20 minutes (Blümcke *et al.*, 1967). There was a reduction in the number of dense-core vesicles, some of which were apparently discharging from the surface of the cells. In this experiment, however, the mitochondria were swollen and the nuclei showed evidence of degeneration suggesting that the changes were not physiological but represented cellular degeneration created by unduly severe hypoxia. Subsequent studies using less severe hypoxia failed to substantiate the findings of Blümcke *et al.* Thus, cats were rendered hypoxic for 45 minutes by administering a mixture of 9 per cent oxygen in nitrogen through an endotracheal tube. (Al-Lami and Murray, 1968). Although the glomic cells of hypoxic cats were more electron-dense than normal, there was no difference in the size, electron density or number of dense-core vesicles. In another study hamsters have also been subjected to atmospheric concentrations of oxygen ranging from 3–5 per cent for 20 minutes (Chen *et al.*, 1969). Subsequent electron microscopy revealed no change in the appearance or numbers of granules in the chief cells or in their cytoplasmic density. Thus, the available evidence suggests that acute exposure to hypoxia does not cause discharge of the dense-core vesicles. This is contrary to what one might expect, since these organelles are believed to contain the catecholamines involved in the chemoreceptor nervous reflex. In this respect the results of experiments with the potent catecholamine-releasing drug reserpine are instructive. In one such experiment massive doses of reserpine were administered to cats (Duncan and Yates, 1967) but failed to produce discharge of the granules in chief cells of the carotid body, despite striking vacuolation of granules in the sympathetic nerve endings and adrenal medulla. Similar results were obtained after reserpine treatment in the hamster (Chen *et al.*, 1969). Interestingly, the nature of the fixative used for electron microscopy influences the observed effect of reserpine. Thus, with osmium tetroxide alone, it reveals a striking reduction in density of the dense-core vesicles, whereas, after fixation in glutaraldehyde followed by osmium tetroxide, no change is observed (Chen *et al.*, 1969; Duncan and Yates, 1967). Since the latter method is a better fixative for protein, it may be that the dense-core vesicles are largely proteinaceous in nature so that depletion of biogenic amines by reserpine causes no structural change in them. The failure of acute hypoxia to induce vacuolation of dense-core vesicles supports this idea or, alternatively, suggests that biogenic amines within the carotid body are not directly involved in the chemosensory reflex (Chen *et al.*, 1969).

Effects of chronic exposure to natural and simulated high altitude

On chronic exposure to the conditions of high altitude, characteristic changes take place in the dense-core vesicles. The first of such studies was that of Edwards *et al.*, (1971) who examined the carotid bodies of guinea pigs which had lived all their lives in Cerro de Pasco, on the Peruvian Altiplano, at an altitude of 14 300 feet (4330 metres) above sea level. Their ultrastructural features were compared with those of sea-level controls. The most striking feature was a pronounced increase in size and vacuolation of the dense-core vesicles (Fig. 6.5). The central dense-core was often reduced in size and density and was excentrically situated in the granule. In some, the core was lost altogether to produce clear vesicles up to 350 nm in diameter. Larger vacuoles, up to 2μm in diameter, were also seen and it was suggested that these may form by progressive dilatation of the clear vesicles or by their fusion (Edwards *et al.*, 1971), thus explaining the vacuolation of chief cells seen in high altitude rabbits and guinea pigs (Chapter 5).

Entirely contrary results were obtained by Møller *et al.*, (1974) who examined the carotid bodies of rabbits living on the Bolivian altiplano at a comparable altitude. These authors described a two-fold increase in the population of dense-core vesicles in the high altitude rabbits, although this figure was obtained purely by subjective impression. Furthermore, the dense-core vesicles were not

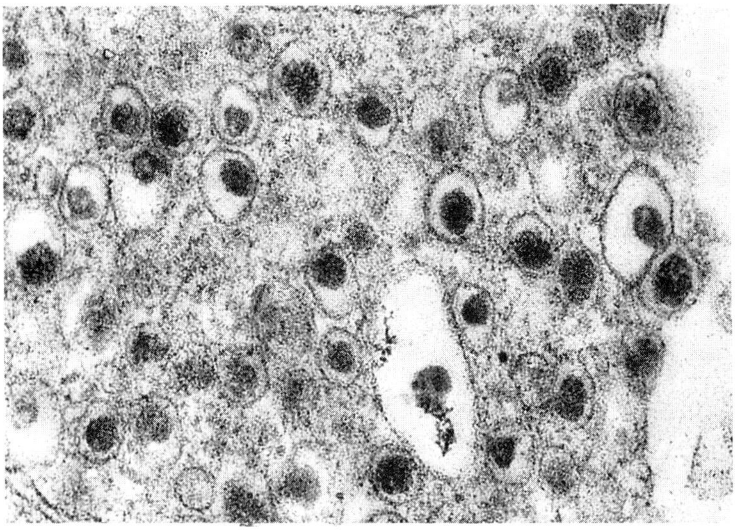

Fig. 6.5 Chief cell from the carotid body of a guinea pig which was born and lived at Cerro de Pasco (4330 m) in the Peruvian Andes. Many of the dense-core vesicles are enlarged with expansion of the clear, peripheral halo. The dense cores are reduced in size and in some granules are pale and indistinct. One granule (*centre*) has enlarged to such an extent as to form a vacuole. (EM × 61 500)

vacuolated in the hypoxic rabbits. A lack of vacuolation of dense-core vesicles was also reported by Blessing and Kaldeweide (1975) in chronically hypoxic rats, but these authors reported a decrease in their numbers.

The findings of Edwards *et al.*, (1971) were supported by further studies on rats which had been kept in a hypobaric chamber, at a simulated altitude of 4300 metres, for four to five weeks (Laidler and Kay, 1978*a*). In this experiment exhaustive measures were taken to exclude autolytic change. In these animals the chief cells of the carotid body showed enlarged, vacuolated dense-core vesicles with excentric cores, as in the guinea pigs from Peru. It is worth noting that similar changes occur in the bronchial Feyrter cell of hypoxic rats (Moosavi *et al.*, 1973). The Feyrter cell has an assumed neuro-endocrine function and an ultrastructure which closely resembles that of the carotid body chief cell.

In order to settle the question as to whether the number of dense-core vesicles changes in response to simulated high altitude Laidler and Kay (1978*b*) extended their studies on rats to include quantitative ultrastructural methods. They found that there was a striking reduction in the number of dense-core vesicles per unit area in test rats. This was, however, associated with a proportionately large increase in cross-sectional area of the whole cell indicating that the total number of granules in each cell was unchanged. There was an overall increase in the number of mitochondria in each cell suggesting an increased metabolic activity. These authors concluded that the chief cells were probably synthesizing more granules than normal but this was balanced by an increased rate of discharge.

Similar changes have not been demonstrated in man, but Arias-Stella and Valcarcel (1973), using formaldehyde-induced fluorescence to demonstrate biogenic amines (Chapter 3), found a reduced reaction in the carotid bodies of Quechua Indians from the Peruvian Andes. This is consistent with a discharge of biogenic amines from the dense-core vesicles but does not indicate whether the proteinaceous core is involved.

The above experiments suggest that vacuolation of dense-core vesicles in animals of natural or simulated high altitude is a genuine structural change rather than an artifact. It is not clear why it has not been demonstrated by all workers, neither is its functional significance known. Although these animals were subjected to the hypoxia of reduced barometric pressure, it is possible that the changes in the dense-core vesicles were not in themselves directly the consequence of hypoxaemia. The loss of the central dense core may represent secretion of a polypeptide hormone in response to one or more of the many other stimuli which occur on chronic exposure to high altitude. For example, man and animals exposed to high altitude show an increased secretion of steroid hormones and it is conceivable that such an endocrine change could initiate alterations in the ultrastructure of chief cells which may themselves be endocrine in nature.

References

Al-Lami, F. & Murray, R.G. (1968). Fine structure of the carotid body of normal and anoxic rats. *Anatomical Record* **160**, 697.

Arias-Stella, J. & Valcarcel, J. (1973). The human carotid body at high altitudes *Pathologia et Microbiologia* **39**, 292.

Blessing, M.H. & Kaldeweide, J. (1965). Light and electron microscopic observations on the carotid bodies of rats following adaptation to high altitude. *Virchows Archives, Abteilung B* **80**, 315.

Blümcke, S., Rode, J. & Niedorf, H.R. (1967). The carotid body after oxygen deficiency *Zeitschrift Zellforschung* **18**, 52.

Chen, I.L., Yates, R.D. & Duncan, D. (1969). The effects of reserpine and hypoxia on the amine-storing granules of the hamster carotid body. *Journal of Cell Biology* **42**, 804.

Duncan, D. & Yates, R. (1967). Ultrastructure of the carotid body of the cat as revealed by various fixatives and the use of reserpine. *Anatomical Record* **157**, 667.

Edwards, C., Heath, D. & Harris, P. (1971). Ultrastructure of the carotid body in high altitude guinea pigs. *Journal of Pathology* **107**, 131.

Jago, R., Smith, P. & Heath, D. (1984). Electron microscopy of carotid body hyperplasia. *Archives of Pathology and Laboratory Medicine* **108**, 717.

Laidler, P. & Kay, J.M. (1978*a*). Ultrastructure of carotid body in rats living at a simulated altitude of 4300 metres. *Journal of Pathology* **124**, 27.

Laidler, P. & Kay, J.M. (1978*b*). A quantitative study of some ultrastructural features of the type I cells in the carotid bodies of rats living at a simulated altitude of 4300 metres. *Journal of Neurocytology* **7**, 183.

McDonald, D.M. & Mitchell, R.A. (1975). The innervation of glomus cells, ganglion cells and blood vessels in the rat carotid body; a quantitative ultrastructural analysis. *Journal of Neurocytology* **4**, 177.

Møller, M., Møllgard, K. & Sørensen, S.C. (1974). The ultrastructure of the carotid body in chronically hypoxic rabbits. *Journal of Physiology (London)* **238**, 447.

Moosavi, H., Smith, P. & Heath, D. (1973). The Feyrter cell in hypoxia *Thorax* **28**, 729.

7. Enlargement in Hypoxaemia

A major cause of enlargement of the carotid bodies is a reduction in the partial pressure of oxygen in the plasma irrespective of whether the causative alveolar hypoxia is environmental or the effect of chronic lung disease. On the other hand, anaemic hypoxia does not lead them to enlarge. The other main cause of an increase in size of the carotid bodies is systemic hypertension (Chapter 8).

Enlargement at high altitude

Enlargement of the carotid bodies in man in hypoxaemia was first reported in native highlanders. In 1969, Arias-Stella reported that the carotid bodies of Quechua Indians living at high altitude in Cerro de Pasco (4330 m), in Central Peru, were larger than those of mestizos dwelling on the coastal plain of that country. This early report was later extended when Arias-Stella and Valcarcel (1973) described the carotid bodies in two series of necropsies; one from mestizos at sea level, and one from Quechuas at 4330 m. The cases were matched for age and sex and mostly comprised accidental deaths with no significant cardiovascular or pulmonary pathology. The cases were compared in the three age groups 10–20 years, 21–40 years and 41–70 years. The carotid bodies of the highlanders were larger and heavier in each age group and the differences became greater with age. While the combined mean weights of the carotid bodies varied very little, from a value of about 25 mg, in the three age groups from sea level, a definitive progressive increment was found with age at high altitude so that in the eldest groups the combined carotid body weight in the highlanders exceeded 60 mg. In this respect it is of interest to recall that physiological studies on the sensitivity of the chemoreceptors at high altitude have been largely in groups of young subjects. It would be worth investigating if the carotid bodies of older highlanders were less sensitive to hypoxia.

Following the original observation of enlargement of the carotid bodies in native highlanders, there were many reports that a similar increase in volume in glomic tissue occurs in domesticated animals living in mountainous areas. Thus enlarged carotid bodies have been reported in guinea pigs, rabbits and dogs (Edwards *et al.*, 1971*a*) and cattle (Arias-Stella and Bustos, 1976). We have already noted in Chapter 5 that the histological appearances of enlarged carotid bodies in different species exposed and acclimatizing to environmental hypoxia are very different from one another (Heath *et al.*, 1985). Furthermore, we recognized there that indigenous mountain animals in contrast have small carotid bodies whose histopathology can be associated with Darwinian adaptation as contrasted to acclimatization (Heath *et al.*, 1985).

Enlargement in pulmonary emphysema

The carotid bodies enlarge in patients with pulmonary emphysema associated with chronic alveolar hypoxia, just as they do in man and domesticated animals living at high altitude (Fig. 7.1). In a study of the post-mortem size and structure

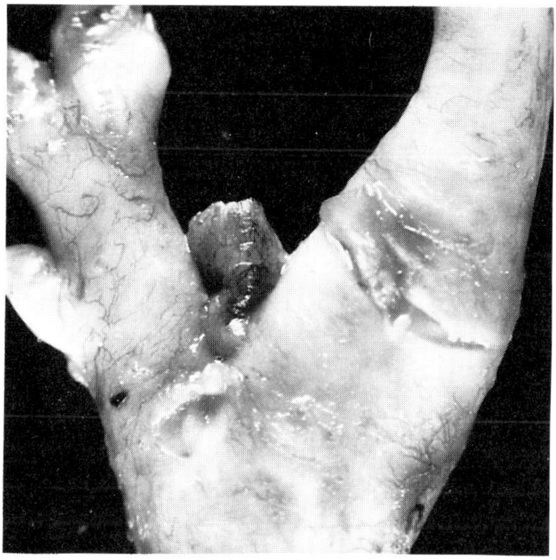

Fig. 7.1 Congested enlarged right carotid body from a man aged 62 years who had panacinar emphysema and left ventricular hypertrophy. Combined carotid body weight in this case was 43.9 mg. (× 3.4)

of the human carotid body at low altitude (Heath *et al.*, 1970) we found that the average weight of the right carotid body was 12.9 mg while that of the left was 11.3 mg, giving a combined weight of 24.2 mg. In two patients with hypoxic cor pulmonale complicating pulmonary emphysema the combined carotid body weight was 60.9 and 68.8 mg respectively, while the combined weight of the carotid bodies in a case of the Pickwickian syndrome was 45.5 mg. In this small group, selected because of the probability of chronic hypoxia having occurred during life, the mean weight of the carotid bodies (58.4 mg) was significantly higher than that of the rest (21.4 mg). The patient with the combined carotid body weight of 60.9 mg was known to have a systemic arterial Po_2 of 36 mmHg and Pco_2 of 54 mmHg during life. These observations were consistent with enlargement of the glomic tissue in response to the chronic hypoxaemia of disease.

In a further series of 44 subjects coming to routine necropsy (Edwards *et al.*, 1971*b*) we point-counted lungs fixed in distension so that the type and severity of any emphysema present could be determined accurately. Thirteen of these cases had no 'significant' emphysema, arbitrarily taken to be 5 per cent or more of centrilobular emphysema or 10 per cent or more of the alveolar duct or panacinar variety, and in them the mean combined weight of the carotid bodies was 21.1 mg. Eleven of the remaining 31 subjects had significant emphysema. In four of these the right ventricular weight was normal and the mean combined carotid body weight was 32.4 mg. In seven of the emphysematous subjects there was right ventricular hypertrophy and the mean combined carotid body weight was 56.2 mg. In one case in this latter group the combined carotid body weight was as high as 89.3 mg. The remaining 20 subjects in this series had systemic hypertension and are considered in Chapter 8.

There was no relation between either the type or the severity of the pulmonary emphysema on the one hand and the weight of the carotid bodies on the other. Clearly then emphysema *per se* does not lead to enlargement of the glomic tissue. Rather there was carotid body enlargement in those cases of emphysema with right ventricular hypertrophy, commonly designated 'hypoxic cor pulmonale'. The factor linking hyperplasia of glomic tissue and right ventricular hypertrophy is almost certainly alveolar hypoxia which leads to hypoxaemia and to muscularization and constriction of the terminal portions of the pulmonary arterial tree elevating vascular resistance. Thus the basic cause of enlargement of the carotid bodies in pulmonary emphysema is the same as that operating in man and animals at high altitude.

Nature of the enlargement in chronic hypoxia

In states of chronic alveolar hypoxia the enlarged carotid bodies show organic changes. In cases of pulmonary emphysema with chronic hypoxaemia and right ventricular hypertrophy one finds the histological picture of numerous small clusters of chief cells surrounded by proliferating sustentacular cells as described in Chapter 5. In native highlanders too, structural changes are found in the carotid bodies. The lobules are larger and more numerous and the collagen bands separating them thinner (Arias-Stella and Valcarcel, 1976). The concentration of parenchymal cells is described as being so dense and diffuse as to give the sections a homogeneous appearance. These authors attempted to measure what they termed 'the functional area' of parenchymal elements. They used one section comprising the entire half surface of the organ from each paraffin block for this purpose. They found that the area occupied by parenchymal cells was significantly greater in native highlanders than in sea-level subjects. Arias-Stella and Valcarcel (1976) described the cells undergoing hyperplasia as chief cells and there was no mention of the proliferation of sustentacular cells which we have found in cases of pulmonary emphysema (Chapter 5). Arias-Stella and Valcarcel (1976) noted that the proliferated chief cells showed depletion of yellow-green, naturally fluorescing, bioamine-containing granules (Chapter 3). The chief cells also showed much cytoplasmic vacuolation. Such changes may have been due to the effects of hypoxia but they could have been due to autolysis, for it is unlikely that material studied on a mountain side, under field conditions, was placed rapidly in the appropriate fixative, as could be achieved under controlled conditions in a laboratory.

Nature of the enlargement in acute hypoxia

In the laboratory, animals may be placed in decompression chambers to simulate the hypobaric hypoxia of high altitude. Under such conditions the carotid bodies may be induced to enlarge but one must be careful to recognize certain features of such experiments that distinguish them from natural exposure to hypoxia as experienced by men living at high altitude or patients suffering from chronic lung disease. In the first case animal experiments are short, lasting a few months, weeks or even days and such acute or sub-acute exposure to hypoxia does not really equate with a lifetime living in the hypoxia of mountains, or years suffering from a chronic lung disease. In the second place our studies of the comparative pathology of the enlarged carotid body (Heath *et al.*, 1985), referred to in Chapter 5, make it clear that the histopathology of carotid body hyperplasia in man is different from that seen in different species of animal. This applies especially to the rat whose glomic tissues appear to be remarkably insensitive to the development of organic changes in response to hypoxaemia.

Bearing in mind these considerations we may now consider the nature of the rapid enlargement of the carotid body that may be induced and equally readily reversed in experimental animals, particularly rats. In one experiment we studied the tissue volume of the carotid body by an application of Simpson's rule (Chapter 1) to histological sections in three groups of 10 adult male Wistar albino rats (Heath *et al.*, 1973). The first group was kept for five weeks in a hypobaric chamber exposed to a barometric pressure of 380 mmHg, equivalent to a simulated altitude of 5500 m above sea level. The second group was exposed to the same barometric pressure for five weeks and then allowed to recover in room air for a further period of five weeks. The third group acted as controls and was kept at normal barometric pressure throughout. In the control animals the mean carotid body volume (expressed in units of $\mu m^3 \times 10^6$) was 13.45, but after exposure to chronic hypoxia for only five weeks this volume rose to 47.81. Once the hypoxic stimulus was withdrawn the tissue volume fell after only five weeks to 19.82. Laidler and Kay (1975) carried out similar morphometric studies on the carotid bodies of rats, some of which had been kept in ambient air at sea level and some of which had been maintained in a decompression chamber at a subatmospheric pressure of 460 mmHg for between 25 and 96 days. They also found a rapid and substantial increase in the volume of the carotid bodies. They expressed their results as combined carotid body volume (i.e. double the values resulting from the experiments of Heath *et al.* (1973) quoted above) and found this to increase from 47.16 in the controls to 187.39 ($\mu m^3 \times 10^6$). They did not find any percentage increase of glomic cells to account for this increase in size. They are of the opinion that such enlargement of the carotid bodies in the rat subjected to acute or subacute hypoxia in a hypobaric chamber is largely due to dilatation of capillaries. This increased vascularity may represent nothing more than a non-specific reaction designed to increase blood flow and thus oxygen transport to the hypoxic organ with increased metabolic activity.

There seems to be no good reason why this rapid enlargement of the carotid body due to vascular engorgement should not take place during the periods of worsening of hypoxaemia that characterize the clinical course of chronic bronchitis and emphysema. Presumably recovery from bouts of superadded chest infections with associated alleviation from hypoxia will also bring about a rapid reversibility of vascular engorgement and a concomitant decrease in size of the carotid body. Chronic exposure to hypoxaemia, however, will in man induce the histological features of carotid body hyperplasia already described in Chapter 5.

Anaemia

The carotid bodies do not enlarge in response to anaemic hypoxia. In one series of cases that we studied we obtained the combined carotid body weights at necropsy in a series of subjects who had been anaemic and related those weights to a representative haemoglobin level measured in the period before death. We studied 26 male and 9 female subjects who had been anaemic and 5 male and 10 female subjects who had not. Criteria for anaemia (de Gruchy, 1972) were taken to be a haemoglobin level below 13.5 g/dl for men and below 11.5 g/dl for women. A wide range of diagnosis accounted for the anaemia in both sexes. The carotid bodies were not enlarged in the subjects who had been anaemic, the mean carotid body weights in the anaemic men and women being respectively 21.8 mg and 13.3 mg, both figures being well within what we regard as a normal range (Chapter 2). Our findings do not confirm the experimental work of Tramezzani and his colleagues (1971) who reported that in cats made chronically anaemic by daily bleeding the carotid bodies enlarged. They also reported that in six cats removal of the carotid bodies led to a fall in the reticulocyte count and to anaemia. Subsequently, Lugliani *et al.* (1977) found no evidence in man of a relation between the carotid bodies and the haemoglobin level, haematocrit reading, or reticulocyte count when they studied a series of patients undergoing bilateral resection of their carotid bodies as part of the treatment of 'chronic obstructive lung disease'. They found there to be no significant change in haematocrit reading or reticulocyte count from preoperative values when studied for a period of up to three years postoperatively. Hence, the results of our study, and those of Lugliani and his colleagues, do not support the suggestion of Tramezzani *et al.* (1971) that the carotid bodies are concerned with the control of erythropoiesis.

References

Arias-Stella, J. (1969). *Human carotid body at high altitudes*. Item 150 in the 69th programme and abstracts of the American Association of Pathologists and Bacteriologists, San Francisco.

Arias-Stella, J. & Bustos, F. (1976). Chronic hypoxia and chemodectomas in bovines at high altitudes. *Archives of Pathology* **100**, 636.

Arias-Stella, J. & Valcarcel, J. (1973). The human carotid body at high altitudes. *Pathologia et Microbiologia* **39**, 292.

Arias-Stella, J. & Valcarcel, J. (1976). Chief cell hyperplasia in the human carotid body at high altitudes. Physiologic and pathologic significance. *Human Pathology* **7**, 361.

de Gruchy, G.C. (1972). *Clinical Haematology in Medical Practice*. Blackwell, Oxford.

Edwards, C., Heath, D., Harris, P., Castillo, Y., Krüger, H. & Arias-Stella, J. (1971*a*). The carotid body in animals at high altitude. *Journal of Pathology* **104**, 231.

Edwards, C., Heath, D., & Harris, P. (1971*b*). The carotid body in emphysema and left ventricular hypertrophy. *Journal of Pathology* **104**, 1.

Heath, D., Edwards, C. & Harris, P. (1970). Post-mortem size and structure of the human carotid body. *Thorax* **25**, 129.

Heath, D., Edwards, C., Winson, M. & Smith, P. (1973). Effects on the right ventricle, pulmonary vasculature, and carotid bodies of the rat on exposure to, and recovery from, simulated high altitude. *Thorax* **28**, 24.

Heath, D., Smith, P., Fitch, R. & Harris, P. (1985). Comparative pathology of the enlarged carotid body. *Journal of Comparative Pathology*, In press.

Laidler, P. & Kay, J.M. (1975). A quantitative morphological study of the carotid bodies of rats living at a simulated altitude of 4300 metres. *Journal of Pathology* **117**, 183.

Lugliani, R., Whipp, B.J., Winter, B., Tanaka, K.R. & Wasserman, K. (1971). The role of the carotid body in erythropoiesis in man. *New England Journal of Medicine* **285**, 1112.

Tramezzani, J.H., Morita, E. & Chiocchio, S.R. (1971). The carotid body as a neuroendocrine organ involved in the control of erythropoiesis. *Proceedings of National Academy of Science USA* **68**, 52.

Winson, M. & Heath, D. (1973). The carotid bodies in anemia. *Archives of Pathology* **96**, 58.

8. Enlargement in Systemic Hypertension

In this chapter we describe the structural changes which occur in the carotid body in systemic hypertension and speculate on their functional significance.

Increase in weight

The weight of the carotid bodies is related to that of the left ventricle. In a series of 15 cases in which the left ventricle weighed more than 200 g, the mean combined carotid body weight was 38.1 mg. Although there was considerable variation in this weight ranging from 17.6–80.8 mg, in 10 instances it exceeded 30 mg. (Edwards *et al.*, 1971). Enlargement of the carotid body in left ventricular hypertrophy appears to be specifically associated with raised intravascular pressure. In 36 cases of systemic hypertension coming to necropsy we weighed the carotid bodies and left ventricle, and found a strongly positive statistical correlation between the two (Smith *et al.*, 1982). The relation is plotted in Figure 8.1, where it will be noted that there was a considerable overlap of carotid body weight between the controls and cases of systemic hypertension, the two groups being separated largely by virtue of their differing left ventricular weights. The mean carotid body weight in the hypertensive group was 30 mg which was statistically significantly different from the mean of 18 mg in the controls, but it was equal to the upper limit of normal. There was also considerable overlap of the 95 per cent probability limits (Table 2.1).

Patients with biventricular hypertrophy due to both pulmonary emphysema and systemic hypertension also have enlarged carotid bodies (Edwards *et al.*, 1971), but the combination of these factors has no additive effect (Fig. 8.1). Myocardial hypertrophy due to valvular defects or cardiomyopathy is in general not associated with carotid body enlargement (Smith *et al.*, 1982), although two cases of aortic stenosis with combined carotid body weights of 39.2 and 40.7 mg have been referred to (Heath *et al.*, 1970).

Histology

The histological features of the carotid body in systemic hypertension are identical to those found in chronic hypoxaemia (Chapter 7) comprising a hyperplasia of elongated cells forming whorls around diminished central cores of chief cells (Smith *et al.*, 1982; Heath *et al.*, 1982) (Fig. 5.1). The lobules are also

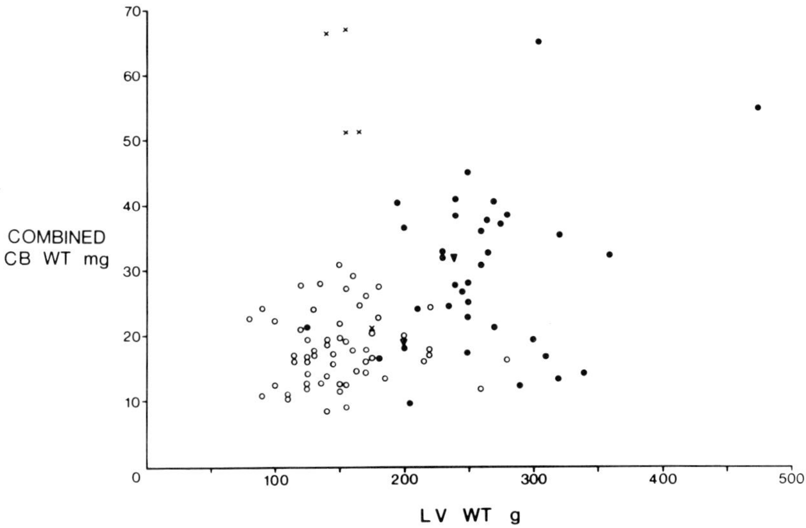

Fig. 8.1 Graph of combined carotid body weight plotted against the weight of the left ventricle. Symbols are the same as in Fig. 3.7. Although the cases with systemic hypertension tend to have heavier carotid bodies, there is considerable overlap with the controls.

increased in size so that in one study of 36 cases the lobule diameter ranged from 272–890μm with a mean value of 581μm (Smith *et al.*, 1982). In individual cases lobules as large as 1500μm may be found (Heath *et al.*, 1982). The mean sustentacular cell count is 54 per cent and when this is plotted against lobule diameter, as in Fig. 3.6, there is a strongly positive correlation between the two (Smith *et al.*, 1982). This graph also includes five cases of hypoxaemia which tend to have larger lobules and more sustentacular cells than the majority of cases of systemic hypertension.

Experimental systemic hypertension

Attempts to elucidate the connection between the carotid body and systemic hypertension have employed the spontaneously hypertensive rat of the Okamoto-Aoki strain. This animal spontaneously develops a severe elevation of systemic arterial blood pressure and is used widely as an experimental model for human systemic hypertension. An elevation of systolic blood pressure occurs at six weeks of age reaching a maximum of 180–220 mmHg by ten weeks (Wong *et al.*, 1982). If the volumes of carotid bodies of these rats are measured by Simpson's rule (Chapter 1) there is an almost three-fold increase over normotensive control rats (Habeck *et al.*, 1981; Honig *et al.*, 1981; Smith *et al.*, 1984). There is no tendency for this enlargement to be progressive so that at 13 weeks of age it is maximal and any subsequent increase in volume is due entirely to growth of the animal (Smith *et al.*, 1984).

Although the carotid body of Okamoto rats is enlarged it is histologically normal. It does not show the vascular engorgement which typifies enlargement of the carotid body in experimental hypoxia (Chapter 5). Neither is there a proliferation of sustentacular cells as in man. In one investigation the hyperplasia was attributed to a proliferation of chief cells (Habeck *et al.*, 1981), on the basis of subjective impression. When we carried out a differential cell count, however, we found that the proportions of chief and sustentacular cells were normal (Smith *et al.*, 1984), suggesting that the enlarged carotid body of the hypertensive rat is produced by proliferation of both types of glomic cell in unison resulting in a normal architecture. This difference in the reaction of the carotid body to systemic hypertension between rats and man suggests that there might also be differences in their physiology. The implication is that the rat is not a good model for the study of carotid body structure and function in man.

An alternative view might be taken that the increased size of the carotid body in Okamoto rats is due not to hyperplasia but to genetic differences between different strains of rat. This is unlikely in view of the fact that in Okamoto rats 5 to 6 weeks old there is already a significant increase in systemic blood pressure but their carotid body volume is normal when related to body weight (Honig, 1983). As the degree of systemic hypertension increases so does the carotid body volume in excess of that in control rats, suggesting that this difference is not genetically determined. Furthermore, the large carotid bodies of Okamoto rats are apparently hyperactive since these animals have a raised partial pressure of oxygen and reduced partial pressure of carbon dioxide in their systemic arterial blood (Przybylski, 1978).

The glomic arteries of Okamoto rats show striking changes which are progressive with age. As early as 13 weeks of age the small muscular arterioles shown an intimal proliferation consisting of dark, elongated cells embedded within a loose matrix. These lesions have been interpreted as consisting of large cells with copious, vacuolated cytoplasm (Habeck *et al.*, 1981). More detailed studies including electron microscopy have shown that the elongated cells are myofibroblasts embedded within a loose matrix of mucopolysaccharide ground substance (Habeck *et al.*, 1983; Smith *et al.*, 1984). These intimal proliferations are lined by plump, basophilic endothelial cells which are sometimes pressed together obliterating the lumen of the vessel. With increasing age of the animal, larger vessels become involved so that by 41 weeks of age the main glomic artery itself may be affected (Smith *et al.*, 1984). There are usually associated changes in the media of affected vessels with fraying of elastic laminae and dilation of a segment of the artery, usually near its origin. It is assumed that the raised systemic pressure dilates and damages glomic arteries and arterioles and the intimal proliferation develops in response to this damage (Smith *et al.*, 1984).

Origin of carotid body hyperplasia in systemic hypertension

It is not easy to explain why systemic hypertension is associated with increased nerve density and secondary proliferation of sustentacular cells in the carotid body. Any explanation offered has to encompass the fact that the same histological changes occur in states of chronic hypoxaemia.

Salt and water retention

It is an intriguing thought that there may be a common physiological link in the three conditions in which we find the most prominent enlargement of the carotid body. These three conditions are ascent to high altitude, pulmonary emphysema, and systemic hypertension. Any lowlander who has visited mountainous areas knows that one of the common dangers of ascent is the retention of sodium and water with the development of the severer forms of acute mountain sickness in the form of high altitude pulmonary or cerebral oedema. It is fascinating that lowlanders who develop enlargement of the carotid body are commonly patients with pulmonary emphysema but only when they begin to retain sodium and water as 'blue bloaters'. These patients certainly have a raised systemic venous pressure and right ventricular hypertrophy but they can hardly be termed to be in cardiac failure since their cardiac output is normal and shows normal exercise tolerance (Harris and Heath, 1977). The increase in extracellular fluid volume which mimics congestive cardiac failure is more likely to be related to disturbed endocrine or renal function. It has been postulated that in systemic hypertension too the primary abnormality may be in the kidney (Poston *et al.*, 1981). It is thus worthy of our attention that hyperplasia of the carotid body seems to occur in those conditions where there is a retention of sodium and water.

This association becomes even more interesting with the recent observation that stimulation of the carotid bodies of animals with hypoxaemic blood results in increased excretion of sodium and water (Honig, 1983). The basis of this natriuresis is uncertain. It could be due to the systemic vasoconstriction and raised systemic arterial blood pressure which follows acute exposure to hypoxia. Such vascular changes might enhance renal perfusion thereby causing an increased excretion of sodium (Honig, 1983) However, this effect is brief and is rapidly followed by a prolonged phase of systemic hypotension. Furthermore, it has to be kept in mind that hypoxia would at the same time induce constriction of renal arteries (Parker, *et al.*, 1975; Bursaux *et al.*, 1976) which would not facilitate renal perfusion.

An alternative view is that it is the carotid body itself which induces the natriuresis. This mechanism might be brought into action to counteract the sodium retention associated with ascent to high altitude, 'blue bloaters', and systemic hypertension. Thus it has been suggested that the defective elimination of sodium in hypertension is being continuously corrected by an increase in concentration of a circulating substance which, by inhibiting sodium reabsorption from the renal tubules, enhances its excretion (Poston *et al.*, 1981).

That such a substance could come from the carotid body has been demonstrated in cats (Honig, 1983; Honig and Schmidt, 1980). They perfused the vascularly isolated carotid bodies of anaesthetised cats with venous blood whilst maintaining a normal circulation of blood in the rest of the body. This hypoxaemic stimulation of the carotid bodies caused an increased rate of breathing and a mild elevation of systemic arterial blood pressure. There was also a significantly raised excretion of sodium in the urine which increased steadily with the duration of hypoxaemia. This reaction was independent of whether or not the vagus nerve was intact, and neither was it related to the raised systemic blood pressure since it still occurred when the renal blood flow was maintained at a constant level (Honig, 1983). In further experiments all neural supply to one kidney was severed and the carotid bodies perfused with hypoxaemic blood as before. The innervated kidney showed vasoconstriction whereas in the denervated one this pressor effect was almost completely abolished thereby demonstrating its isolation from the nervous system. Nevertheless, there was still an increased excretion of sodium from the denervated kidney (Honig and Schmidt, 1980). These experiments suggest a reflex control of renal tubular sodium absorption which is independent of a neural supply and which may, therefore, be mediated by a circulating substance or hormone originating from the carotid body. In chronic hypoxaemia or systemic hypertension the tendency to retain sodium and water may lead to a chronically increased demand for this substance thereby causing the carotid body to become hyperplastic.

Baroreception and chemoreception

It would appear that these two functions are intimately connected in some way in this specialized vascular area at the carotid bifurcation. An increase in systemic arterial blood pressure enhances the chemosensory reflex. Thus, in young men with early, mild systemic hypertension, there is physiological evidence of increased sensitivity of their chemoreceptors (Trzebski *et al.*, 1982) with a higher than normal minute ventilation breathing normal air (Quies *et al.*, 1983). Similarly, in young, spontaneously hypertensive rats, there is a raised Pa_{O_2} and a decreased Pa_{CO_2} suggestive of hyperventilation (Przybylski, 1978). This enhanced chemoreceptor activity in hypertensive rats is persistent (Honig, 1983). Clearly, enhancement of the chemosensory reflex could result by direct stimulation, by raised intravascular pressure or by involvement of the carotid body or central nervous system. Our findings of enlargement of the carotid body in systemic hypertension in men and Okamoto rats suggests that in some way glomic tissue is involved. However, at present, we cannot explain why this enlargement should be associated with differential hyperplasia or nerve axons and supporting sustentacular cells in man but not in the spontaneously hypertensive rat.

The carotid body as baroreceptor

Classical physiological theory teaches that the carotid body is concerned with chemoreception and the carotid sinus with baroreception but our argument above leads us to the interesting concept that the carotid body may act also as baroreceptor. We shall see in the following chapter (Chapter 9) that some of its arteries have a structure very similar to that of the carotid sinus which we consider in Chapter 12 and which is classically regarded as the baroreceptor of the body. Thus, the media of the main glomic artery is thin and consists of tightly-packed elastic fibres with little intervening smooth muscle, showing a remarkable similarity to the carotid sinus (Jago *et al.*, 1982). Like the sinus, the main glomic artery is richly supplied by nerve axons, although it is not known if these are cranial or autonomic in origin. Some of the branches of the main glomic artery also have this peculiarly thin-walled elastic structure which is so different from that of arteries of similar calibre elsewhere in the systemic circulation. All of this suggests that the highly-elastic, thin walls of parts of the glomic arterial tree has a specific functional connotation, perhaps that of baroreception. One could postulate that in man, but not in the Okamoto rat, the increased axonal density and secondary supportive hyperplasia of sustentacular cells, represents a response to sustained stimulation of these baroreceptors. At first sight this would not seem to indicate why an identical proliferation of nerve axons and sustentacular cells occurs in states of chronic hypoxaemia. There may, however, on further consideration of this problem be a link in the concept of ischaemia of glomic tissue.

Ischaemia of the carotid body

Systemic hypertension may lead to obstruction of the glomic vessels and hence to ischaemia of the carotid bodies (Quies *et al.*, 1983; Habeck *et al.*, 1983). This may cause the glomic tissue to respond in the same manner as it does to chronic hypoxaemia. Certainly, the glomic arteries of spontaneously hypertensive rats show progressive narrowing by an intimal proliferation of myofibroblasts and mucopolysaccharide ground substance (Habeck *et al.*, 1983; Smith *et al.*, 1984). Also, the glomic arteries of hypertensive patients show an extensive intimal proliferation of fibroelastic tissue, sometimes associated with hyaline change in the media (Habeck *et al.*, 1983; Quies *et al.*, 1983). It has even been argued that congenital thickening of the orifices of glomic arteries actually induces systemic hypertension (Przybylski, 1981) but against this is the obvious fact that increased intravascular pressure in Okamoto rats precedes vascular lesions and carotid body hyperplasia (Honig, 1983). The intimal fibrosis and narrowing of glomic arteries is a prominent feature of ageing in the human carotid body and it too is sometimes associated with proliferation of sustentacular cells.

References

Bursaux, E., Poyart, C. & Bohn, B. (1976). Renal hemodynamics and renal 0_2 uptake during hypoxia in the anaesthetized rabbit. *Pflügers Archives* **365**, 213.

Edwards, C., Heath, D. & Harris, P. (1971). The carotid body in emphysema and left ventricular hypertrophy. *Journal of Pathology* **104**, 1.
Habeck, J.O., Honig, A., Pfeiffer, C. & Schimdt, M. (1981). The carotid bodies in spontaneously hypertensive (SHR) and normotensive rats — a study concerning size, location and blood supply. *Anatomischer Anzeiger (Jena)* **150**, 374.
Habeck, J.O., Waller, H. & Protze, J. (1983). Pathological alterations of the arterial vessels of the carotid bodies in hypertensive humans. *Deutsche Gesundheitswesen (Berlin)* **38**, 1970.
Harris, P. & Heath, D. (1977). *The Human Pulmonary Circulation* (Second Edition). Churchill Livingstone, Edinburgh.
Heath, D., Edwards, C. & Harris, P. (1970). Postmortem size and structure of the human carotid body. *Thorax* **25**, 129.
Heath, D., Smith, P. & Jago, R. (1982). Hyperplasia of the carotid body. *Journal of Pathology* **138**, 115.
Honig, A. (1983). Role of the arterial chemoreceptors in the reflex control of renal function and body fluid volumes in acute arterial hypoxia. In: *Physiology of the Peripheral Arterial Chemoreceptors*, (pp. 395-429). Eds: H. Acker and R.G. O'Reagan. Biomedical Press: Elsevier/North Holland.
Honig, A., Habeck, J.O., Pfeiffer, C., Schmidt, M., Huckstorf, C., Rotter, H. & Eckermann, P. (1981). The carotid bodies of spontaneously hypertensive rats (SHR): A functional and morphological study. *Acta Biologica et Medica Germanica* **40**, 1021.
Honig, A. & Schmidt, M. (1980). Kidney function during carotid chemoreceptor stimulation. Influence of unilateral renal nerve section. In: *Hormonal Regulation of Sodium Excretion* Eds: B. Lichardus, R.W. Schrier and J. Ponec. Biomedical Press: Elsevier/North Holland.
Jago, R., Heath, D. & Smith, P. (1982). Structure of the glomic arteries. *Journal of Pathology* **138**, 205.
Parker, P.E., Dabney, J.M., Scott, J.B. & Haddy, F.J. (1975). Reflex vascular responses in kidney, ileum and forelimb to carotid body stimulation. *American Journal of Physiology* **228**, 46.
Poston, L., Sewell, R.B., Wilkinson, S.P., Richardson, P.J., Williams, R., Clarkson, E.M., MacGregor, G.A. & de Wardener, H.E. (1981). Evidence for a circulating sodium transport inhibitor in essential hypertension. *British Medical Journal* **282**, 847.
Przybylski, J. (1978). Alveolar hyperventilation in young spontaneously hypertensive rats. *IRCS Medical Science (Cardiovascular System)* **6**, 315.
Przybylski, J. (1981). Do arterial chemoreceptors play a role in the pathogenesis of hypertension? *Medical Hypotheses* **7**, 127.
Quies Von, W., Claus, T. & Honig, A. (1983). Die Hyperventilation der Hypertoniker, — Eine Pilotstudie zum Verhalten der Reflexe der arteriellen chemorezeptoren bei hypertensiven Erkerankungen. *Deutsche Gesundheitswesen (Berlin)* **16**, 612.
Smith, P., Jago, R. & Heath, D. (1982). Anatomical variation and quantitative histology of the normal and enlarged carotid body. *Journal of Pathology* **137**, 287.
Smith, P., Jago, R. & Heath, D. (1984). Glomic cells and blood vessels in the hyperplastic carotid bodies of spontaneously hypertensive rats. *Cardiovascular Research* **18**, 471.
Trzebski, A., Tafil, M. Zoltowski, M. & Przybylski, J. (1982). Increased sensitivity of the arterial chemoreceptor drive in young men with mild hypertension. *Cardiovascular Research* **16**, 163.
Wong, G.W.K., Melax, H., Singh, D.N.P. & Jeria, M.J. (1982). Ultrastructural myocardial degeneration in spontaneously hypertensive rats under chronic saline intake. *IRCS Medical Science (Cardiovascular System)* **10**, 155.

9. The Glomic Vasculature

The carotid body receives a rich blood supply from one or more glomic arteries which arise typically from the external carotid artery a few millimetres distal to the bifurcation, although they may originate occasionally from other sites (Chapter 2). The blood flow through the carotid body is very large in relation to its small size and some authorities consider that a considerable proportion of it reaches the glomic veins without having passed through the glomic capillaries (Joels and Neil, 1963). The glomic blood vessels have been far more extensively studied in animals than in man but the account given here is based on the human carotid body. Their unusual histological features suggest that they are more than passive conveyors of blood. The effects of occlusion of the small radicles of the glomic arteries are of interest to the pathologist and we consider these in Chapter 8. The glomic arterial tree comprises the main trunk with its first-order branches, and a system of branches within the substance of the carotid body consisting of interlobular arteries, intralobular arterioles, precapillaries and capillaries (Fig. 9.1). Glomic veins form a diffuse plexus of indeterminate origin.

The main glomic artery

The main glomic artery is ensheathed by the fibrous tissue of Mayer's ligament which also contains the sinus nerve. It is a short vessel estimated as being 1 to 2 mm long in one study (Heath and Edwards, 1971) and 3.5 to 4 mm in another (Jago *et al.*, 1982). The luminal diameter of its free portion is in the region of 200 μm. Despite its small diameter the main glomic artery retains the structure of an elastic vessel which is more typical of large systemic arteries such as the common carotid artery (Jago *et al.*, 1982). At its origin it is encircled by closely-packed bands of thick elastic fibres derived from the parent vessel. In man there are no sphincters guarding its orifice (Jago *et al.*, 1982) in contrast to what is found in the rat (McDonald and Larue, 1983).

Soon after its origin the media of the glomic artery becomes thin and consists of closely adjacent elastic fibres arranged circumferentially. There is virtually no smooth muscle between them and the few cells present are largely fibrocytes (Jago *et al.*, 1982). The histological appearances are reminiscent of those of the carotid sinus suggesting that the glomic artery may subserve a similar baroreceptor function. Exceptionally one may find glomic arteries with concentric elastic laminae widely separated by bundles of circularly and longitudinally orientated smooth muscle cells (Heath and Edwards, 1971).

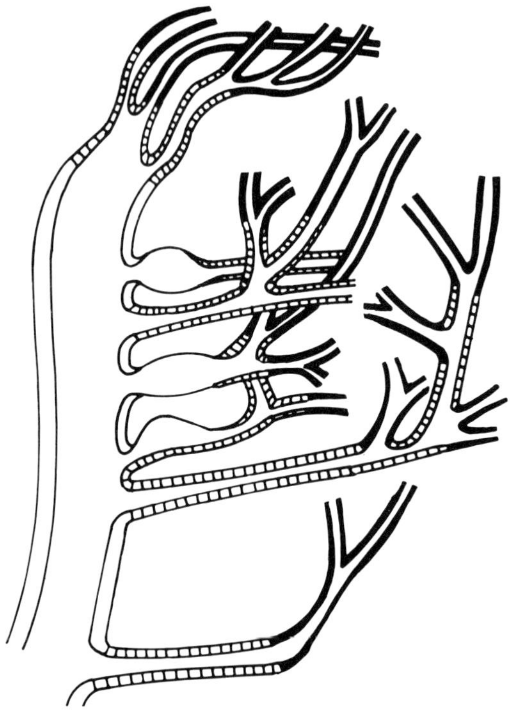

Fig. 9.1 Diagrammatic, two-dimensional representation of the glomic vasculature of the left carotid body of a man of 23 years who died from a cerebellar haemorrhage. The diagram was constructed from serial histological sections stained by the elastic Van Gieson technique. A branch of the main glomic artery is unshaded; interlobular arteries are cross-hatched; intralobular arterioles are black.

The ultrastructure of the free portion of the glomic artery closely resembles that of the carotid sinus (Jago *et al.*, 1982). Thus, in both vessels there is a single layer of endothelial cells resting upon a basal lamina of amorphous ground substance containing fine collagen fibrils. The media of both vessels consists of broad elastic fibres woven into skeins forming a series of layers encircling the artery. The spaces between successive elastic fibres are narrow and contain scanty cells comprising largely fibrocytes with a few, finely attenuated smooth muscle cells. These are associated with ground substance, collagen fibres and small fragments of elastin. Non-myelinated nerve axons are commonly encountered throughout the media of both vessels but, in the case of the main glomic artery in man, the nature and connections of these nerves has not yet been established.

It is of interest to note that the arteries supplying glomic tissue elsewhere in the body also develop the same elastic structure immediately before coming into close approximation with the glomus. Thus, the vessels supplying the mediastinal glomera are branches of the coronary artery and have the typical histological structure of muscular systemic arteries. However, in the immediate vicinity of glomic tissue they undergo an abrupt transition into elastic vessels. Having passed the glomus they revert back to the expected muscular appearance (Edwards and Heath, 1970). Vessels supplying the aorticopulmonary glomus on the dorsal surface of the pulmonary trunk, erroneously termed the 'glomus pulmonale' (Chapter 11), also show the same elastic structure (Edwards and Heath, 1969).

Shortly before reaching the carotid body the glomic artery usually divides into two or three first-order branches (Fig. 9.1) which enter the substance of the organ. The media of these vessels still retains an elastic structure but is considerably thicker than the media of the free portion. Their elastic laminae vary greatly in thickness from coarse, well-defined fibres to short wisps of elastin (Fig. 9.2). These fibres are more widely separated than in the free portion of the vessel with sparsely distributed smooth muscle cells between them. Nevertheless, the histological appearance remains very much a predominantly elastic structure (Fig. 9.2).

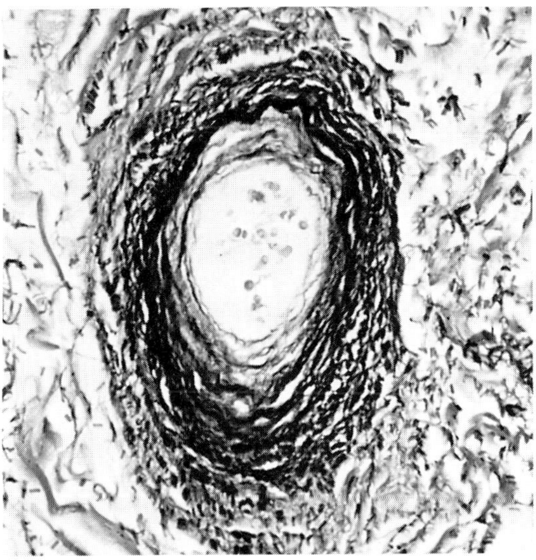

Fig. 9.2 A first-order branch of the main glomic artery in a woman of 80 years who died from ischaemic heart disease. The media consists almost entirely of concentric rings of elastic tissue of variable thickness. There is also moderate fibrosis of the intima associated with ageing. (Elastic Van Gieson × 220)

Interlobular arteries

The main glomic artery and its first-order branches give rise to arterial branches which extend between the lobules of glomic tissue (Fig. 9.1). Because of their location they are best termed interlobular arteries (Heath *et al.*, 1983). They range in external diameter from 150 to 75μm and their media shows an irregular arrangement of anastomosing elastic fibres which are of variable thickness and present a ragged appearance (Fig. 9.3). Between the elastic fibres are numerous smooth muscle cells which are orientated circumferentially. There is no clearly-defined external lamina to these vessels so that the elastic fibres of the media tend to merge with those in the connective tissue of the adventitia (Fig. 9.3). In this way the histological appearance differs markedly from the media of solid smooth muscle that would be anticipated in the typical systemic artery of this diameter.

Their ultrastructure too is irregular and distinct from that of most other systemic arteries. Thus, the prominent elastic laminae are arranged in the form of a net, which divides the media into compartments (Heath *et al.*, 1983). Within the individual compartments are isolated smooth muscle cells, orientated

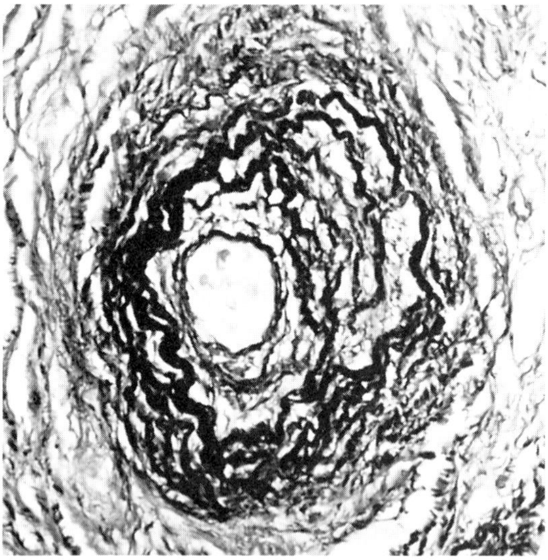

Fig. 9.3 Interlobular artery from the same case. The media is ill-defined and its borders merge into the fibrous tissue of the intima and adventitia. It consists of irregular, anatomosing elastic fibres separating bundles of smooth muscle cells. (EVG × 330)

circularly in the main, and a haphazard arrangement of collagen fibres. Nerve axons are plentiful, usually embedded within the bundles of elastic and collagen fibres (Heath *et al.*, 1983). Isolated smooth muscle cells may also be found within the intima and adventitia so that the limits of the media become indistinct.

The medial thickness of interlobular glomic arteries varies widely over short distances. In some sections it may occupy more than 20 per cent of the external diameter (Heath *et al.*, 1983) whereas in a nearby section it may be extremely thin (Fig. 9.4). Thin segments of interlobular arteries are most commonly found close to their origin, and may involve their whole circumference or only part of it (Fig. 9.4). The media of these thin portions consists merely of a few beaded elastic laminae compressed tightly with no discernible smooth muscle between them. The diameter of the vessel is often greater than elsewhere so that there may be a resemblance to a miniature carotid sinus (Fig. 9.1). It is conceivable that these thin regions are focal baroreceptors.

Intralobular arterioles

The arterial vessels which enter the lobules of glomic tissue (Fig. 9.1) are predominantly muscular and thus more closely resemble systemic arterioles elsewhere (Fig. 9.5). These intralobular arterioles are extremely small with an external diameter ranging from 75 to 15μm (Heath *et al.*, 1983). At their origin there is sometimes a focal pad of smooth muscle cells resembling an arterial ring or blocking mechanism. It is possible that such structures function as arteriolar sphincters.

The media of intralobular arterioles consists of a thick ring of circularly orientated smooth muscle fibres sandwiched between internal and external elastic laminae. Even in these small vessels the elastic tissue is deposited irregularly, often showing discontinuities, fraying and branching (Fig. 9.5), and

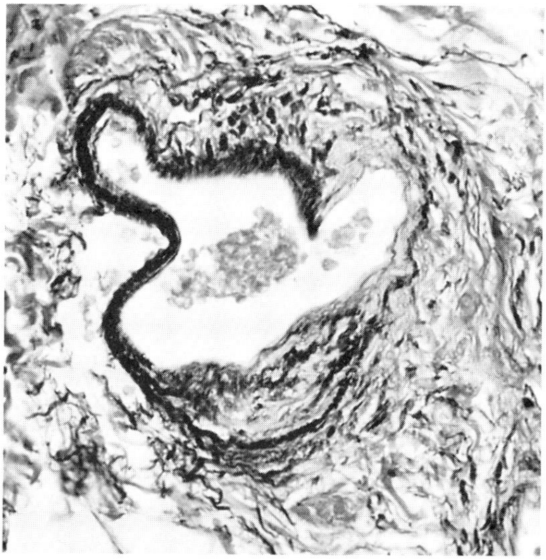

Fig. 9.4 Interlobular artery from a woman of 46 years with a cerebral astrocytoma. The section is from near the origin of the vessel and shows extreme thinning of part of its circumference. In this region the elastic laminae are tightly pressed together with no intervening smooth muscle. (EVG × 300)

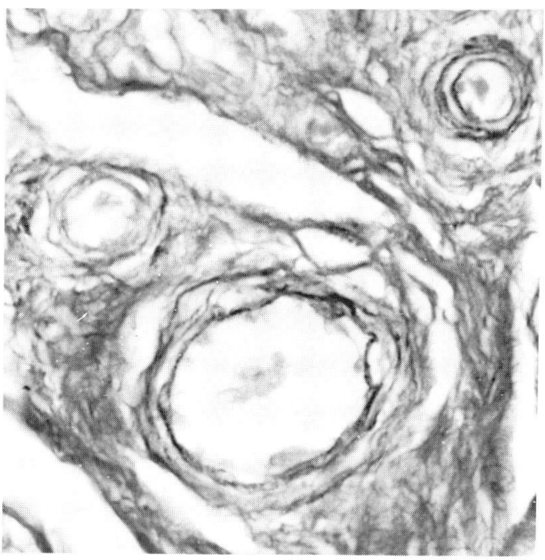

Fig. 9.5 Three intralobular arterioles of differing calibre from a man of 28 years with non-Hodgkin's lymphoma. The vessels consist of a media of circularly orientated smooth muscle with distinct internal and external elastic laminae. The largest arteriole shows focal swellings and protuberances in its media. (EVG × 600)

in some vessels may suggest a spiral configuration. There is considerable variation in the quantity of elastic tissue present in arterioles from different carotid bodies so that in some the arterioles are clearly defined (Fig. 9.5), whereas in others they may require close examination to identify them. The media of some glomic arterioles show focal areas of thickening producing bulbous prominences of the elastic laminae (Fig. 9.5). In some of the smallest radicles of the arteriolar system these focal thickenings may be prominent and pale. Nuclei may be found within them but frequently they appear to be completely empty (Fig. 9.6). Electron microscopy has shown that some of them correspond to enlarged smooth muscle cells with distension of mitochondria

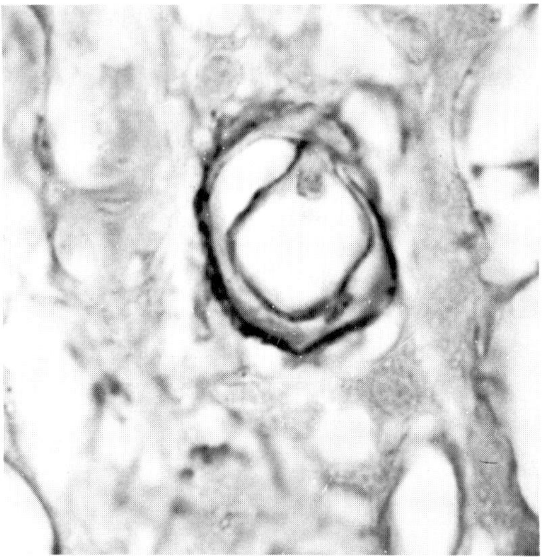

Fig. 9.6 Transverse section of an intralobular arteriole showing areas of pallor in its media producing a variable thickness. (EVG × 1500)

attributed to autolysis. Others correspond to increased amounts of tissue fluid separating the smooth muscle from the internal elastic lamina (Heath *et al.*, 1983). Such focal areas of pallor may, therefore, be artifactual but it is not known why they should occur in the carotid body and not other organs.

Precapillaries and capillaries

Intralobular arterioles undergo a gradual transition into precapillaries in which the internal elastic lamina followed by the media is gradually lost. Transitional forms with an incomplete media may be seen (Heath *et al.*, 1983). Precapillaries consist of a single elastic lamina internal to which is a thin layer of fibroelastic tissue lined by endothelial cells. They extend from the arterioles, which are situated between cell clusters, into the clusters themselves. Here they lose all their elastic tissue and become capillaries which are of the fenestrated type (Chapter 4).

Glomic capillaries are sometimes referred to as sinusoids but this is a misnomer, since all vascular channels in the carotid body are lined by endothelium. Capillaries follow a tortuous path through the cell clusters which is impossible to trace using conventional histological sections. It requires serial reconstructions of sections 1 μm thick to determine their pathway. Using this technique on rats McDonald and Larue (1983) identified two types of capillary. Type I capillaries are the most numerous with a large diameter (8 to over 20 μm), a thin endothelium and a tortuous course amongst the chief cells. These correspond to the so-called 'sinusoids' typical of man. Type II capillaries are narrower in diameter (6 μm) and thus resemble capillaries of striated muscle. They take a more direct route from precapillaries to venules and are less intimately associated with chief cells, often skirting around the perimeter of cell clusters. Their endothelium is thicker and is surrounded by more pericytes than type I capillaries. Both types are preceded by precapillary sphincters. It is not known whether there are type II capillaries in human carotid bodies.

Glomic capillaries come into close juxtaposition with chief and sustentacular cells over approximately half their circumference. The remainder contacts stromal elements. This unit comprising a capillary with its small group of closely adjacent glomic cells is assumed to be the smallest functional unit in the carotid body. It has been termed a 'glomoid' (Seidl, 1975).

Intimal fibrosis

Glomic arteries commonly show an irregular intimal proliferation of collagen together with variable amounts of fine elastic fibrils (Fig. 9.2). This intimal proliferation is often excentrically situated and of variable thickness along the vessel. It appears to become commoner and more pronounced with advancing age in common with the other arteries throughout the body. It seems to be exaggerated in the presence of systemic hypertension (Chapter 8).

Pattern of branching

The manner in which the glomic arteries divide and ramify throughout the carotid body can be studied by corrosion casting of the vasculature followed by scanning electron microscopy (McDonald and Larue, 1983; Seidl, 1975) or by reconstruction of serial sections (McDonald and Larue, 1983; Heath *et al.*, 1983). The human carotid body is sufficiently large to examine corrosion casts with a dissecting microscope. They reveal that, in addition to the main glomic artery, there are usually one, or occasionally two, accessory glomic arteries arising from separate sites on the artery of origin (Fig. 9.7). Supernumerary glomic arteries have also been noted in serial sections (Heath and Edwards, 1971). Both the main glomic artery and accessory arteries continue for a few millimetres towards the carotid body without branching but, just before entering its substance, each divides into an average of three (Fig. 9.7). These first-order branches diverge to the peripheral aspect of the organ where they give rise to numerous lateral branches. Further division is best studied by reconstruction of serial sections an example of which is shown in Figure 9.1. This diagram shows a first-order branch of the main glomic artery passing through the connective tissue in the periphery of the carotid body. It gives rise to several interlobular arteries from its inner aspect which arise at right angles and traverse the connective tissue septa between lobules. The origins of some of these tributaries are dilated and thin-walled as described above. Interlobular arteries may themselves divide or terminate directly as muscular intralobular arterioles which penetrate the lobules of glomic tissue. Note that some arterioles are short whereas others continue for some considerable distance before ending as precapillaries.

Towards the upper pole of the carotid body the first-order branches of the

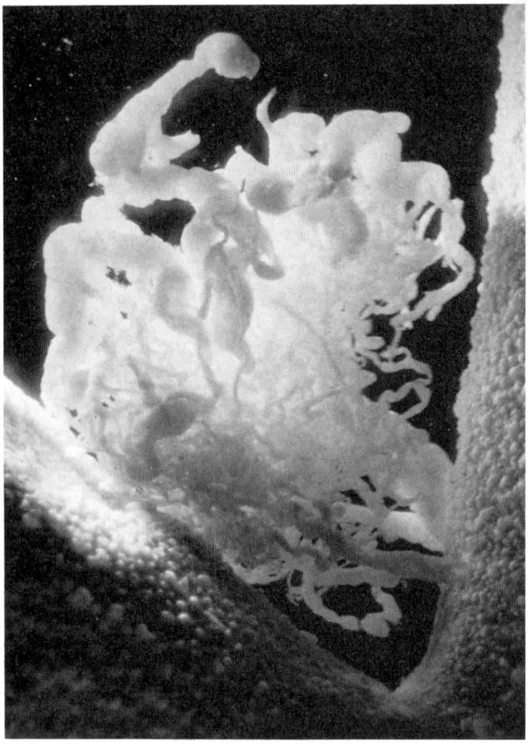

Fig. 9.7 Corrosion cast of the glomic vasculature in a normal carotid body. The main glomic artery arises from the external carotid artery. A smaller, subsidiary glomic artery arises from a separate location in front of it. Both vessels divide into three branches. The large convoluted vessels at the upper pole are glomic veins.

glomic artery narrow until they adopt the structure of interlobular arteries (Fig. 9.1). They then leave their peripheral position and enter the interlobular septa giving rise to the several intralobular arterioles (Fig. 9.1). Thus all the branches of the main glomic artery terminate eventually as precapillaries within the glomic tissue.

Glomic veins

The capillaries of the carotid body drain into venules but the precise point at which this transition occurs is difficult to determine. Venules are thin-walled vessels which form a tortuous series of dilated channels lined by endothelium ramifying through the glomic lobules. These drain into larger venules within the interlobular septa which then run radially to form the tributaries of small veins in the fibrous capsule (Heath *et al.*, 1983). There are numerous veins within the capsule which form a plexus enclosing the entire organ. At the upper pole, this venous plexus becomes more concentrated as large veins are encountered (Fig. 9.7). Thus unlike the polarized arterial supply, the venous drainage is profuse and occupies the entire surface of the carotid body.

Arteriovenous anastomoses

There is some doubt as to whether arteriovenous anastomoses exist in the human carotid body, although they have been demonstrated in animals. Thus physiologists have shown that the blood flow through the carotid body of the cat is 40μl per min corresponding to a flow of 2000 ml per min per 100 g of tissue (Daly *et al.*, 1954). This is extremely high being roughly five times the blood flow in the kidney or four times that in the thyroid (Joels and Neil, 1963). The carotid body of the cat also has an exceptionally high oxygen consumption (Purves, 1970*a*) but, despite this, there is a negligible arteriovenous oxygen difference during normal blood flow (Daly *et al.*, 1954). A small oxygen difference can be measured when the blood flow is drastically reduced. These observations led physiologists to propose that much of the blood from the carotid body artery by-passes the glomic capillaries through arteriovenous anastomoses (Joels and Neil, 1963; Purves, 1970*b*; Acker and O'Reagan, 1981). Joels and Neil (1963) calculated that, if all the blood entering the carotid body were to pass through the capillaries, the oxygen tension could never be reduced sufficiently to initiate a chemosensory reflex dependent on hypoxia. In order for this to occur, three quarters of the blood must be diverted away from the glomus cells, presumably through arteriovenous anastomoses (Joels and Neil, 1963).

Such anastomoses were demonstrated in the carotid body of the cat by de Castro (1951). He observed the carotid bodies in this species *in vivo* during ventilation with different gas mixtures. Hypoxia caused a decrease in their size with an associated reddening due to increased surface blood flow. With a high oxygen content in the inspired air the carotid body became paler and swelled and this was associated with a reduction in venous outflow. De Castro concluded that in cats peripheral arteriovenous shunts are normally operating diverting blood from the glomus cells, but in hypoxia there is an increase in this shunt rendering the cells even more hypoxic. De Castro also performed carmine-gelatin injection studies to demonstrate these anastomoses which he found linking glomic arterioles with veins. These anastomoses have also been shown in the cat by corrosion casting and dye injection studies (Schäfer *et al.*, 1973; Seidl, 1975). In the dog, wide-bore terminal branches of the glomic artery end in thick-walled arterioles, but some pass directly into veins in the periglomic connective tissue (Serafini-Fracassini and Volpin, 1966). The glomic arterioles may end either as capillaries or as anastomotic channels connecting small veins. Minute arteriovenous anastomoses have also been demonstrated in the rat (McDonald and Larue, 1983; McDonald and Haskell, 1984). These are only 10μm in diameter and require careful reconstruction of thin serial sections to detect them. It should be pointed out, however, that some of the first order branches of the carotid body artery of the rat do not supply the carotid body and, those which do, emerge at its distal pole to supply other organs.

There is no convincing evidence that similar anastomoses exist in man. Nothing is known of the oxygen consumption and blood flow of the human carotid body so that theoretical considerations of Joels and Neil cannot be applied. By examination of serial sections from human necropsies we have failed to reveal any direct communication between glomic arteries or arterioles and glomic veins (Heath *et al.*, 1983). Indeed, as shown in Fig. 9.1 all the radicles of the first order branches of the glomic artery terminate as intralobular arterioles which then appear to adopt the structure of precapillaries. Anastomoses of smaller calibre than arterioles may exist as in the rat, but would escape detection by standard serial histological sections. Alternatively, if the anastomoses passed well clear of the carotid body, they would not appear on the sections at all. Corrosion casts, however, do not reveal the existence of such widely-diverging anastomoses (Fig. 9.7).

References

Acker, H. & O'Reagan, R.G. (1981). The effects of stimulation of autonomic nerves on carotid body blood flow in the cat. *Journal of Physiology (London)* **315**, 99.

Daly, M. de B., Lambertsen, C.J. & Schweitzer, A. (1954). Observations on the volume of blood flow and oxygen utilization of the carotid body in the cat. *Journal of Physiology (London)* **125**, 67.

de Castro, F. (1951). Sur la structure de la synapse dans les chemorecepteurs: leur mecanisme d'excitation et rôle dans la circulation sanguine locale. *Acta Physiologia Scandinavica* **22**, 14.

Edwards, C. & Heath, D. (1969). Microanatomy of glomic tissue of the pulmonary trunk. *Thorax*, **24**, 209.

Edwards, C. & Heath, D. (1970). Site and blood supply of the intertruncal glomera. *Cardiovascular Research* **4**, 502.

Habeck, J.-O., Waller, H. & Protze, J. (1983). Pathological alterations of the arterial vessels of the carotid bodies in hypertensive humans. *Deutsche Gesundheitswesen (Berlin)* **38**, 1970.

Heath, D. & Edwards, C. (1971). The glomic arteries. *Cardiovascular Research* **3**, 303.

Heath, D., Jago, R. & Smith, P. (1983). The vasculature of the carotid body. *Cardiovascular Research* **17**, 33.

Jago, R., Heath, D. & Smith, P. (1982). Structure of the glomic arteries. *Journal of Pathology* **138**, 205.

Joels, N. & Neil, E. (1963). The excitation mechanism of the carotid body. *British Medical Bulletin* **19**, 21.

McDonald, D.M. & Haskell, A. (1984). Morphology of connections between arterioles and capillaries in the rat carotid body analysed by reconstructing serial sections. In: *The Peripheral Arterial Chemoreceptors*. Ed: D.J. Pallot. Croom Helm, London.

McDonald, D.M. & Larue, D.T. (1983). The ultrastructure and connections of blood vessels supplying the rat carotid body and sinus. *Journal of Neurophysiology* **12**, 117.

Purves, M.J. (1970*a*). The effect of hypoxia, hypercapnia and hypotension upon carotid body blood flow and oxygen consumption in the cat. *Journal of Physiology (London)* **209**, 395.

Purves, M.J. (1970*b*). The role of the cervical sympathetic nerve in the regulation of oxygen consumption of the carotid body of the cat. *Journal of Physiology (London)* **209**, 417.

Schäfer, D., Seidl, E., Acker, H., Keller, H.-P. & Lübbers, D.W. (1973). Arteriovenous anastomoses in the cat carotid body. *Zeitschrift Zellforschung* **142**, 515.

Seidl, E. (1975). On the morphology of the vascular system of the carotid body of cat and rabbit and its relations to glomus Type I cells. In: *The Peripheral Arterial Chemoreceptors*. Ed: M.J. Purves. Cambridge University Press, London and New York.

Serafini-Fracassini, A. & Volpin, D. (1966). Some features of the vascularization of the carotid body of the dog. *Acta Anatomica* **63**, 571.

10. Chemodectomas

As we have seen in Chapter 1 the carotid body shares identical histological features with other glomera scattered widely throughout the body. While neither the carotid body nor their closely-related glomera strictly fulfil the criteria for designation as non-chromaffin paraganglia some authorities like Glenner and Grimley (1974) are prepared to accept tumours arising from them as non-chromaffin paragangliomas. Although we prefer not to accept this concept for the reasons outlined in Chapter 1, we recognize the close histological resemblance and, thus, after we have discussed the tumour of the carotid body we shall consider very briefly the neoplasms arising from some of the other glomera. This has a certain practical importance for in dealing with a carotid body tumour associated with a nodule of similar histological appearance elsewhere in the body the pathologist has to decide if this represents a metastasis from the carotid body tumour or a second primary arising independently from one of the other glomera (Conley, 1965). In this respect, carotid body tumours have been reported in association with tumours arising in the ganglion nodosum or in one of the aortic arch bodies (Lattes, 1950), with bilateral tumours of the organ of Zuckerkandl (Cragg, 1934) and with a phaeochromocytoma (Cone, 1958).

The chemodectoma

Some early authors used the totally non-committal term of 'carotid body tumour' and there is still much to recommend this simple designation which avoids all controversy over such terms as non-chromaffin paraganglioma. In 1950, Mulligan coined the term 'chemodectoma' in recognition of the characteristic function of chemoreception by the carotid body. This designation has been widely accepted and we shall use it here. Chemodectomas form fairly smooth globular or ovoid tumours between 2.0 to 4.0 cm (Pryse-Davies *et al.*, 1964) and 7.5 cm (Wilson 1966) in diameter (Fig. 10.1). Rarely, tumours as large as 15 cm in diameter (Glenner and Grimley, 1974) have been reported. On section the tumour presents a firm, resilient cut surface which varies in colour from pink-grey to red-brown. There is a fibrous capsule which may be wide or ill-defined. When a chemodectoma is received as a surgical specimen, it will commonly show tags and adhesions of fibrous tissue which represent the connective tissues densely binding it to the adventitia and wall of the carotid artery. Such a

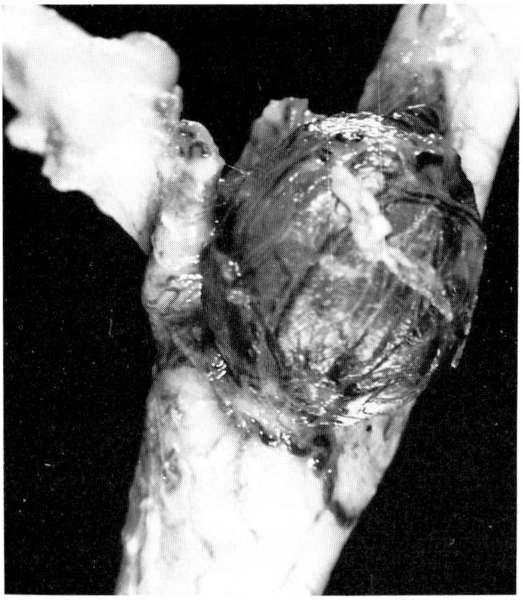

Fig. 10.1 Chemodectoma in a woman of 74 years with systemic hypertension. (× 3.4)

specimen will also commonly show the grooving produced by the closely adjacent and adherent arteries at the site of the carotid bifurcation where it was growing (Pryse-Davies *et al.*, 1964).

Clinical features

Chemodectomas may present at any age. In a series of 90 patients with carotid body tumours seen at the Mayo Clinic during the period 1931 to 1967 the age of presentation ranged from 12 to 63 years (Shamblin *et al.*, 1971). There is no sex preponderance. The chemodectoma presents as a slowly growing firm mass in the neck which earned the old surgical description of 'the potato tumour'. Since it is fixed to the carotid arteries it does not move with swallowing and will move laterally but not vertically. In the Mayo Clinic series the initial complaint of all but one of the patients was that of a mass growing in the neck. One of these patients had bilateral tumours and in a further six subjects a second chemodectoma developed later on the contralateral side. Similarly, all but two of the 41 patients reported by Lees *et al.* (1981) presented to a clinician on account of a mass in the neck which was increasing in size. These tumours grow very slowly. In the series of Shamblin *et al.* (1971) a lump in the neck had been present on average for 6.6 years before the patient presented for surgery and, in one instance, it had been noticed for no less than 47 years. It is worthy of note that no fewer than 19 of the 90 patients reported that there had been a noticeable increase in size in the tumour in the six months before examination. Usually the swelling is said not to be tender on palpation. Pain from the tumour is exceptional.

As we have seen in Chapter 9 the carotid body is a highly vascular structure and in a minority of cases this high blood flow causes the tumour to pulsate and develop a murmur and bruit (Javid *et al.*, 1976). This high blood flow is utilized in the diagnosis of chemodectomas through the agency of angiography. Masses which may be confused with chemodectomas are lymph nodes enlarged due to involvement by lymphoma, tuberculosis or metastases from a thyroid carcinoma. Other masses which have to be distinguished from carotid body tumours are pleomorphic salivary adenomas, neurofibromas, branchial cysts, aneurysms of the carotid artery, and arteriovenous fistulas. Only half of the patients have other symptoms. Headache is a common but non-specific symptom which could have a psychological basis. Hoarsensess, or vocal cord or hypoglossal paralysis are occasionally seen (Javid *et al.*, 1976; Lees *et al.*, 1981) but care must be taken that any cranial nerve involvement noted is not ascribed to the tumour when in fact it may be due to previous surgery. Dizziness, and tinnitus or hearing loss have also been recorded (Javid *et al.*, 1976; Shamblin *et al.*, 1971).

Familial incidence

It has been known for a long time that this tumour tends to show a familial incidence (Chase, 1933; McNealy and Hedin, 1939; Lewison and Weinberg, 1950). The genetic transmission is most consistent with autosomal dominance (Glenner and Grimley, 1974). The largest family group involved was that described by Sprong and Kirby (1949) with eleven siblings; tumours of the neck were known to have occurred in nine members of this family and been surgically resected in six. Katz (1964) reported a family in which three members had bilateral carotid body tumours.

Endocrine activity

Since the first description of a noradrenaline-secreting carotid body tumour by Glenner *et al.* (1962) other functioning tumours of this type have been described (Berdal *et al.*, 1962; Fries and Chamberlin, 1968; Hamberger *et al.*, 1967). Grimley and Glenner (1967) point out that, although most of these tumours were at or near the carotid bifurcation, they were also intimately attached to the cervical sympathetic chain near the superior cervical ganglion. The first reported tumour contained high levels of noradrenaline (1.5 mg/g of tumour) and was associated with clinical findings characteristic of phaeochromocytoma.

Histology

The chemodectoma tends to reproduce some histological features of the normal carotid body. In particular it shows appearances more or less akin to the classical cell clusters or 'zellballen' (Fig. 10.2). However, a range of histological appearances may be presented by these tumours according to the size of the

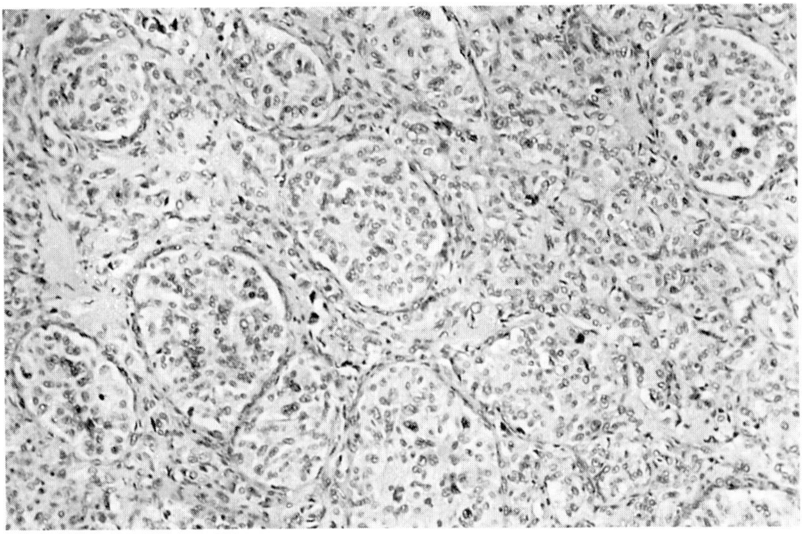

Fig. 10.2 Benign chemodectoma showing characteristic zellballen. (HE × 120)

neoplastic cell clusters. In some the clusters are large and well-defined (Fig. 10.2) and are delineated by fine reticulin fibres which present a most characteristic pattern as a network of boxes. These reticulin fibres are easily picked out by silver stains (Chapter 3) and sometimes form denser, thicker bands. They do not penetrate between individual tumour cells.

The tumour cells themselves appear to be derived from chief cells (Chapter 3) and have typical open round or oval nuclei, 5 to 12 μm in diameter, with a moderate chromatin content and occasional prominent nucleoli. The margins of the cells cannot be distinguished clearly and they present a palely eosinophilic, syncytial appearance. The cytoplasm may show fine vacuolation. Electron microscopy of these closely-applied cells may reveal intercellular adhesions which in fact correspond to the puncta adherentia of normal chief cells and which resemble the desmosomes or tight junctions of epithelial tissues. Hence the presence of desmosomes in a tumour queried as a chemodectoma should not be taken as proof that it is in fact a tumour of epithelial origin.

Not all chemodectomas have this classical alveolar pattern of well-defined, large clusters of pale chief cells enclosed in their individual box outlined by reticulin fibres. In many tumours the neoplastic cell clusters are very small and, if their organization into these separate units is not recognized, could be interpreted as sheets of epithelial cells (Fig. 10.3). The plump chief cells have abundant pale cytoplasm and give an impression of hypercellularity. Occasional, well-defined and sizeable 'zellballen' may occur within these expanses of neoplastic mini-clusters. A characteristic feature of the chemodectoma is the presence of broad bands of relatively acellular fibrous tissue staining palely with eosin. We refer to these fibrous trabeculae further below. Not infrequently one finds the combination of sheets and strands of neoplastic mini-clusters

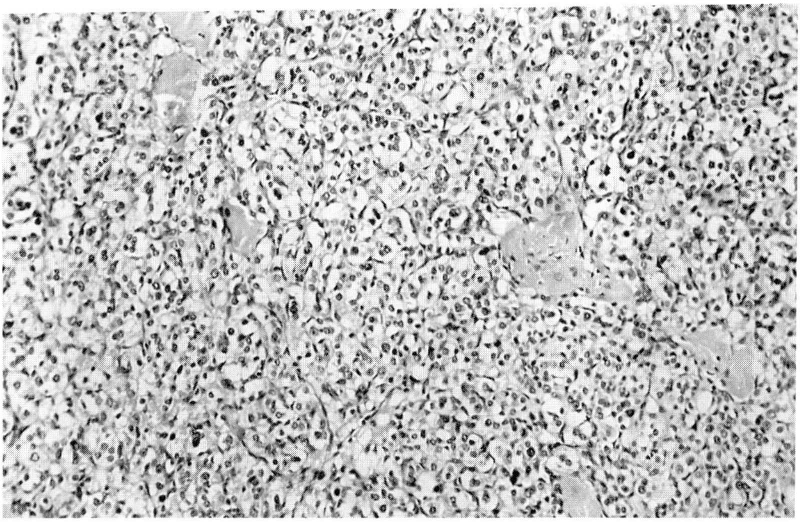

Fig. 10.3 Benign chemodectoma from a woman of 56 years showing a micro-alveolar form in which the clusters are so small as to suggest sheets of epithelial cells. (HE × 120)

infiltrating these broad bands of fibrous stroma. Dilated sinusoid-like vascular channels are sometimes seen and these may isolate individual cell clusters into discrete bands. Sometimes one has the impression that haemorrhage has occurred into cell clusters and may be the origin of some of these vascular spaces which appear to be lined directly by neoplastic chief cells without intervening endothelium.

Glenner and Grimley (1974) believe that there are differences in the cytoplasmic density in the cells of a chemodectoma which correspond to that of light and dark variants of chief cells described in Chapter 3. They say that this distinction can be made out particularly when the cytoplasmic processes of adjoining light and dark cells interdigitate with one another. Such interdigitation is seen well in thin, plastic sections of tumour fixed well in glutaraldehyde. It is, however, far more difficult to make out in routine paraffin sections.

Sometimes the clusters of chief cells are surrounded by a rim of more elongated cells which might represent sustentacular cells (Pryse-Davies *et al.*, 1964; Grimley and Glenner, 1967). Some chemodectomas are said to be composed entirely of spindle-shaped cells (Grimley and Glenner, 1967) but we think that, when sheets of elongated cells are found, the possibility of malignancy must be considered, as described below. Rarely, anastomosing cords of elliptical or spherical cells are encountered mimicking the trabecular pattern of some morphological varieties of functioning adrenal medullary phaeochromocytoma.

Carotid body tumours are usually non-chromaffin but occasionally cytoplasmic granules in individual or small groups of cells will exhibit chromaffinity (Pryse-Davies *et al.*, 1964). This is probably due to catecholamines (Chapter 3) but could be due to lipochrome pigment which is sometimes found. Some chemodectoma cells will show the yellow-green colour of formalin-induced fluorescence which is also consistent with the presence of catecholamines. Fluorescence and tissue assay for catecholamines are useful for diagnostic purposes.

Various types of granule can be demonstrated in chemodectoma cells. Many are reduced by the Masson-Fontana and del Rio Hortega silver methods. Such argentaffin reactions in carotid body tumours have been studied extensively (Barroso-Moguel and Costero, 1962; Costero and Barroso-Moguel, 1961; Costero and Chevez, 1962). Intracellular glycogen is not present and the cells do not react with the periodic acid-Schiff stain. As noted above, lipochrome may occasionally be found; such pigments are found in some chief cells in the normal carotid body (Chapter 3). They stain with oil red O and take up azo dyes but Schmorl's reaction is negative. Small haemorrhagic foci are sometimes found in chemodectomas so that deposits of haemosiderin are common. Various enzyme activities of a non-specific nature have been demonstrated by Pryse-Davies *et al.* (1964). Arylesterase ('non-specific esterase') activity of a type seen in normal paraganglia and ganglion cells may be demonstrated in most chief cells of the tumour. The tumour cells show moderate acid phosphatase activity whilst the cells lining the sinusoid-like vessels show alkaline phosphatase activity. Lactic and succinic dehydrogenase activity is generalized in tumour and stromal cells (Pryse-Davies *et al.*, 1964).

Usually received with a surgical specimen of chemodectoma is a variable amount of fibrous tissue beyond the confines of the tumours and within this may be found arteries, veins, myelinated and non-myelinated nerves, ganglion cells and small collections of lymphocytes, plasma cells and mast cells. Any of these components may also on occasion be found within the stromal regions of the tumour itself but the normal relation of nerve fibres to chief cells is not seen in chemodectoma thus providing evidence that it is truly neoplastic and not a hamartoma (Grimley and Glenner, 1967). The superficial layer of fibrous tissue and its contained vascular channels may extend into the tumour in trabecular fashion. Within the tumour these vessels soon come to comprise little more than an endothelial lining supported by delicate reticulin fibres and they may on occasion be so numerous as to suggest that the tumour is angiomatous in nature. A pronounced hyaline change may occur in the fibrous tissue around the vessels (Glenner and Grimley, 1974).

One of the characteristic histological features of the chemodectoma is its tendency to show nuclear pleomorphism, even in tumours which are unequivocally benign on clinical grounds (Fig. 10.4). There may be considerable variation in size and shape of the chief cells. Hyperchromatic nuclei and bi- and tri-nucleate cells may be found but mitotic figures are exceedingly rare. Even a large giant cell with a single nucleus may be discovered, although this may represent a surviving ganglion cell (Pryse-Davies *et al.*, 1964). Such appearances

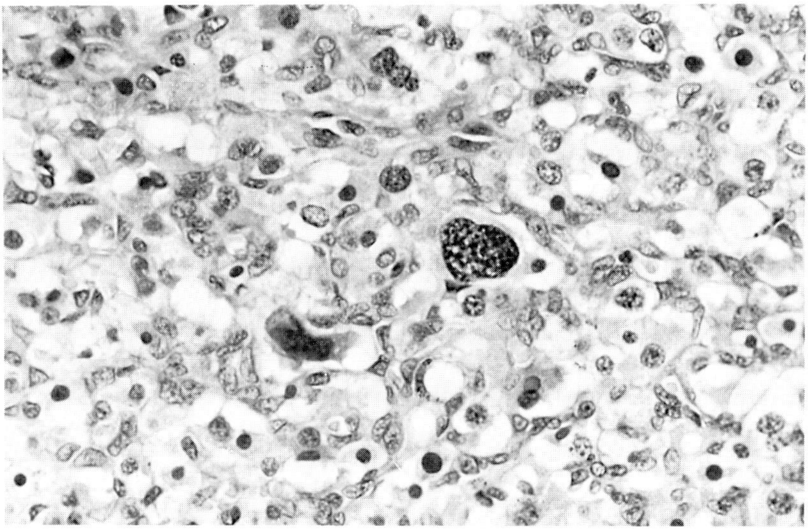

Fig. 10.4 Benign chemodectoma from a woman of 48 years showing cellular pleomorphism. (HE × 375)

may be disturbing but the histopathologist must be on his guard against accepting such appearances as indicators of malignancy. Nevertheless, undoubted malignant change with local or distant spread does occur in the chemodectoma. We must consider this difficult problem now.

Malignant change

Local invasion of the wall of the carotid arterial bifurcation occurs in about 5 per cent of cases but metastasis to regional lymph nodes and distant viscera also takes place. Shamblin and his colleagues (1971) believe that the assertion of malignancy must rest on such spread. In 500 cases of chemodectoma reported up to that year they found sixteen (about 3 per cent) with local infiltration, and sixteen with distant metastasis. Hence the reported incidence of malignancy was about 6 per cent. Staats *et al.* (1966) had previously given the same percentage of local and distant malignancy. There is an extensive bibliography authenticating metastasis of chemodectoma to lymph nodes or viscera and a few illustrative papers are those of Donald and Crile (1948), Goormaghtigh and Pattyn (1954), Romanski (1954), Turnbull (1954), Morfit *et al.* (1953), Westbury (1963), Rabson and Elliot (1957), Fanning *et al.* (1963), Gustilo *et al.* (1965), and Reese and Bergman (1963). The lungs and skeleton are especially susceptible to metastasis (Brown *et al.*, 1967).

As we have noted above, prediction of the behaviour of a chemodectoma from its histological appearance is difficult, if not impossible. Cellular and nuclear pleomorphism and hypercellularity are not uncommon features of benign tumours. Glenner and Grimley (1974) examined several malignant carotid body tumours and found that they showed hyperchromatic nuclei with variation in size and shape with large nucleoli but significantly these nuclear abnormalities appeared no more frequently than in benign lesions. Multinucleated giant cells and mitotic figures, although very rare, have been reported in carotid body tumours but they are not reliable indices of malignancy (Pryse-Davies *et al.*, 1964). Shamblin *et al.* (1971) reported a series of cases of chemodectoma from the Mayo Clinic and this included two cases that had metastasized; in neither instance was there any histological evidence of malignancy. A patient of Lees *et al.* (1981) showed the histological features of a benign chemodectoma and yet subsequently exhibited widespread lymphatic metastasis. Romanski (1954) carefully compared two clinically malignant chemodectomas with five benign tumours and was unable to detect histological differences from which the differing biological behaviour could have been predicted. Le Compte (1951) was of the opinion that even the occurrence of chemodectoma cells within blood vessels does not seem to be a valid criterion of malignancy. Brown and his colleagues (1967) have pointed out that there may be a long interval up to 35 years between observation of the primary tumour and occurrence of metastatic lesions.

In Figures 10.5 and 10.6 we illustrate histological features of a malignant chemodectoma which occurred in a man of 70 years. Cell clusters delineated by reticulin fibrils are still clearly seen (Fig. 10.5). There is, however, a striking

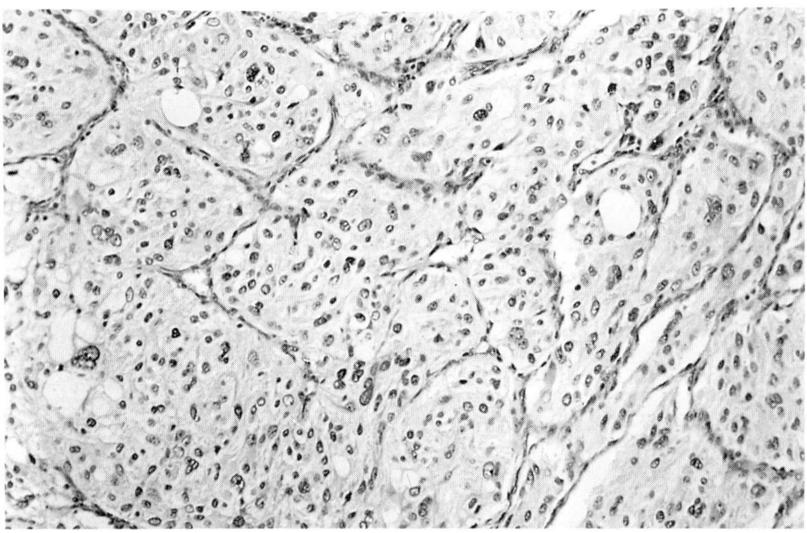

Fig. 10.5 Malignant chemodectoma from a man of 70 years. Zellballen are still clearly visible but there is considerable cellular pleomorphism. (HE × 120)

degree of cellular and nuclear pleomorphism (Fig. 10.5). The cytoplasm of the cells of some of the neoplastic clusters is brightly eosinophilic and the margins of such clusters are particularly indistinct and infiltrative (Fig. 10.6). In other neoplastic cell clusters the cytoplasm has remained faintly eosinophilic. Many

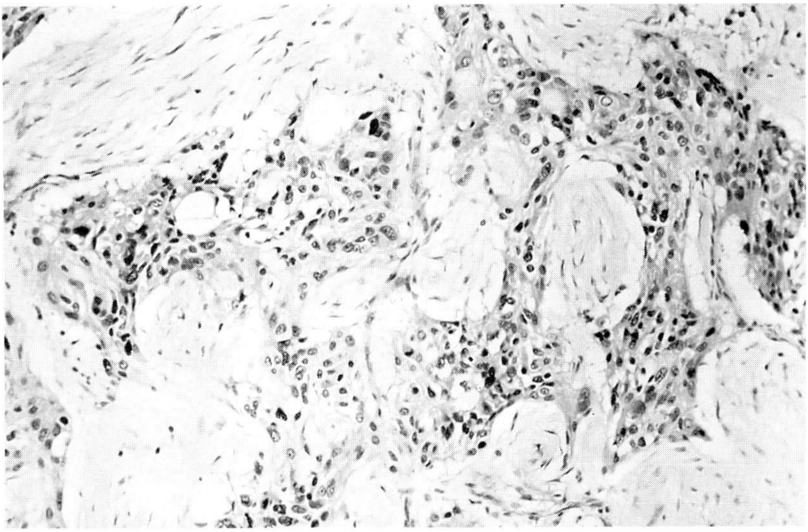

Fig. 10.6 Malignant chemodectoma from the same case illustrated in the preceding figure. This area of the tumour shows striking eosinophilia and pleomorphism. (HE × 120)

of these clusters show a streaming of elongated cells into the surrounding tissue (Fig. 10.6). Hence in this case the two histological features that distinguished the case from a benign chemodectoma were the great variations in two cell populations with regard to the eosinophilia of their cytoplasm and the development of sheets of infiltrative, spindle-shaped cells. Two years later this chemodectoma, which was unequivocally malignant on histological grounds, metastasized to regional lymph nodes. The histology of the metastasis was the same as that of the primary tumour with areas of infiltrative eosinophilic tumour and sheets of elongated cells. The cases we have illustrated in the necessarily restricted number of figures in this chapter show the two extreme histological situations ranging from unequivocally benign (Figs 10.2 to 10.4) to undoubtedly malignant (Figs 10.5 and 10.6). However, it has to be accepted that there are many intermediate cases where the detection of malignant change is very difficult. Under such circumstances it is imperative for the pathologist to be cautious when advising the surgeon or patient on prognosis.

Electron microscopy

A suspected diagnosis of chemodectoma can usually be confirmed by electron microscopy since the neoplastic cells retain many of the ultrastructural features of the normal carotid body, including the striking dense-core vesicles (Fig. 10.7). However, the technique will not distinguish between a carotid body tumour and a vagal paraganglioma since both have an identical fine structure (Kahn, 1976). Even if the resected tissue is fixed in glutaraldehyde immediately after surgical

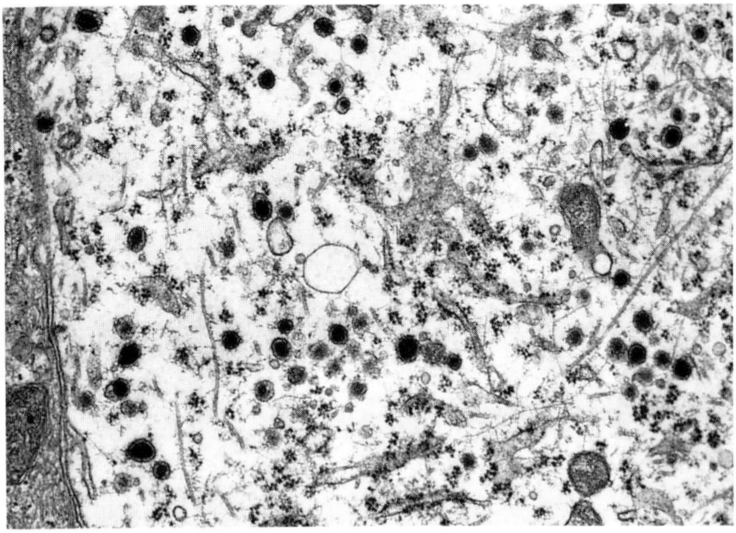

Fig. 10.7 Electron micrograph of chemodectoma showing the characteristic dense-core vesicles. (EM × 23 400)

removal, preservation of cellular detail may be poor owing to the prolonged ischaemia which occurs during dissection. Nevertheless, cellular organelles are usually sufficiently intact to be recognizable. Resected tissues fixed in formalin may show severe cellular degeneration on electron microscopy, but even using such tissue it commonly proves possible to identify the dense-core vesicles and hence recognize the tumour as a chemodectoma.

At the ultrastructural level, the chemodectoma comprises two main components, rounded clumps of chief cells separated by a vascular stroma. Unlike the normal organ the chief cells at the edge of the clumps may come into direct contact with fenestrated capillaries (Grimley and Glenner, 1967; Capella and Solcia, 1971). Most chief cells closely resemble those of the normal carotid body in that they are polygonal with large, pale nuclei and contain numerous mitochondria, variable amounts of smooth and rough endoplasmic reticulum and dense-core vesicles (Toker, 1967; Grimley and Glenner, 1967; Alpert and Bochetto, 1974; Robertson and Cooney, 1980). Cell junctions resembling desmosomes may be found occasionally between chief cells, but in malignant chemodectomas such junctions are extremely rare (Robertson and Cooney, 1980). It has already been pointed out that puncta adherentia are a normal feature of chief cells and hence the demonstration of desmosome-like structures should not be taken as an indication that the tumour is epidermal in nature.

Although the chief cells are polygonal in the main, some may give rise to long, highly attenuated processes or else the entire cell may be elongated. In many chemodectomas light and dark variants of chief cells can be recognized largely by virtue of their cytoplasmic density (Grimley and Glenner, 1967; Alpert and

Bochetto, 1974; Robertson and Cooney, 1980). This distinction is, however, not as clear-cut as in the normal organ and a continuous spectrum of cytoplasmic density may be present instead (Robertson and Cooney, 1980).

The organelles most typical of the chemodectoma, as in the normal carotid body, are the dense-core vesicles. In most carotid body tumours these vesicles are of the same size and configuration as normal (Fig. 10.7) but a variable degree of pleomorphism may be encountered such as two distinct populations of granules, one large and one small (Toker, 1967; Alpert and Bochetto, 1974) or tubular and dumb-bell forms (Robertson and Cooney, 1980). Several authors describe the presence of occasional cells in which dense-core vesicles are sparse and the cytoplasm is filled instead with numerous, enlarged mitochondria reminiscent of the oncocytes of endocrine tumours (Grimley and Glenner, 1967; Capella and Solcia, 1971; Robertson and Cooney, 1980).

Sustentacular cells and nerve axons are not features of chemodectoma. Elongated cells are frequently found at the periphery of the clumps of chief cells and have been referred to as sustentacular (Alpert and Bochetto, 1974) but they often contain dense-core vesicles and are thus highly attenuated chief cells (Toker, 1967; Capella and Solcia, 1971; Robertson and Cooney, 1980). This paucity of sustentacular cells might be expected since nerve axons are rare or absent from chemodectomas (Toker, 1967; Alpert and Bochetto, 1974; Grimley and Glenner, 1967; Robertson and Cooney, 1980). The peripheral, elongated chief cells often contain numerous residual bodies and lipofuscin granules.

Metastases of malignant chemodectomas have the same ultrastructural appearances as the primary tumour (Robertson and Cooney, 1980). It should be borne in mind, however, that the presence of dense-core vesicles in metastatic tumours does not necessarily distinguish them from other malignant glomus tumours or from the carcinoid tumour (Bensch *et al.*, 1965). In this situation, positive identification depends upon locating the primary neoplasm.

Prevalence at high altitude

Chemodectomas occur more frequently in man and cattle living at high altitude. Arias-Stella and Bustos (1976) claimed that as many as 40 per cent of cattle living at an elevation of 4330 m in the vicinity of Cerro de Pasco in the Andes of Central Peru develop histological changes in their carotid bodies suggestive of chemodectoma. All but two of 25 Peruvian adults with chemodectomas of the head and neck studied by Saldaña and his colleagues (1973) had been born and lived at altitudes between 2105 and 4350 m above sea level, whereas only 38 per cent of the Peruvian population of 13.5 million live at or above an altitude of 3000 m (Peruvian Census, Monge, 1966). This suggests that the carotid body tumour is ten times more frequent at high altitude than at sea level. In their series of 23 cases they found that all the carotid body tumours in their patients were benign apart from one malignant glomus jugulare tumour. Females predominated over males by about six to one and left-sided tumours were three times more prevalent. Histologically, the tumour cells were arranged in clusters and comprised chief cells in which the dark variety predominated. This increased prevalence of chemodectoma has been reported only in two species both of which have to acclimatize to the hypobaric hypoxia of high altitude. It has not been described in animal species like the llama and alpaca which show a genetic Darwinian adaptation to life to the high mountains. Saldaña *et al.* (1973) thought that the very slow rate of growth of these tumours and their benign clinical course were consistent with their being hyperplastic rather than frankly neoplastic in nature.

Influence of chronic lung disease

Chedid and Jao (1974) reported the occurrence of 11 tumours of the carotid body and one chemodectoma of the ganglion nodosum of the right vagus nerve in six members of two consecutive generations of a family. All affected members had bilateral tumours of the carotid bodies with a single exception. No fewer than four of these six patients had associated chronic obstructive pulmonary disease with a persistently high systemic arterial Pco_2 and low Po_2 levels. One case of bilateral carotid body tumour reported by Saldaña *et al.* (1973) occurred in a 29-year-old Indian man at 3870 m who had worked as a miner for 12 years and developed silicosis. In this case the combined effects of the hypoxia of lung disease and high altitude appear to have formed a powerful stimulus to chemodectoma formation.

Association with thyroid carcinoma

Albores-Saavedra and Durán (1968) reported the association of chemodectoma with thyroid carcinoma in two patients in Mexico City (2380 m). In these cases the carcinomas were of papillary and follicular type in contradistinction to the medullary carcinoma of the thyroid which occurs in association with phaeochromocytoma. Both the carotid body and the adrenal medulla share a common origin from neural ectoderm and a common function in secretion of catecholamines. Two of the patients from the Andes with chemodectomas reported by Saldaña and Salem (1970) and Saldaña *et al.* (1973) also died of metastasizing thyroid carcinoma.

Treatment

The features of chemodectomas that influence treatment are their unusual position closely adjacent to major arteries and the demonstration that about 6 per cent of them will progress to local invasion or distant metastasis. Previously many surgeons believed that chemodectomas were always benign and slow-growing and, as removal was difficult, it was thought best to leave well alone. A more recent school of thought thinks that the potentially invasive nature of the tumour requires a more aggressive surgical approach (Javid *et al.*, 1976). This is best carried out when the tumour is small and its excision carries less morbidity. This emphasizes the importance of accurate diagnosis by carotid angiography at an early stage. Diagnostic angiography will usually reveal an extremely vascular tumour supplied by one of the arteries of the carotid bifurcation. There may be splaying of the internal and external carotid arteries. Larger lesions may require sacrifice of the external carotid artery with replacement of the arterial defect with a vein graft. A definitive operation for a carotid body tumour is carried out only after a previous diagnostic exploration or a biopsy in up to a third of cases (Browse, 1982). Not uncommonly it is misdiagnosed as an enlarged cervical lymph node and discovered by a young, inexperienced surgeon attempting a biopsy, sometimes under local anaesthesia.

The position of the chemodectoma between the origins of the internal and external carotid arteries may make the surgical resection of the tumour very difficult. According to Browse (1982), 'No surgeon should attempt to remove a carotid body tumour unless he is experienced in the surgical technique used for carotid artery surgery for atheromatous disease. This means that any surgeon who finds such a tumour unexpectedly should stop the operation, without a biopsy, and arrange for the patient to have further investigations and re-exploration by an experienced vascular surgeon. To proceed unprepared with excision without the correct vascular instruments and surgical skill is hazardous and might cause a stroke — an unacceptable complication of what the patient had probably been told was to be a simple biopsy of a node'. In most cases the tumour can be removed without damaging the carotid artery by dissecting within the adventitia. The dissection is always bloody but the oozing stops as soon as the tumour is free. Sometimes the tumour is so intimately adherent to the walls of the carotid arteries that it is difficult to remove without making a hole in the adjacent vessels.

Local invasion of the vascular wall occurs in about 5 per cent of cases and this may mean that the tumour must be removed *en bloc*. For this to be done safely the cerebral circulation has to be maintained with a shunt and the excised vessel replaced with a reversed autogenous graft of saphenous vein. The impossibility of predicting whether or not this major procedure will be necessary must restrict performance of the operation to vascular surgeons. Nowadays, under such conditions the risk of stroke should be minimal. The other risk is damage to the hypoglossal or vagus nerves resulting in an awkward tongue or a husky voice.

Shamblin and his associates (1971) reported the results of surgery for chemodectoma performed at the Mayo Clinic over the period 1931 to 1967. Their report illustrates that in the early years before the advent of modern vascular surgical techniques there was a significant post-operative morbidity associated with the removal of these tumours including damage to the carotid arterial tree with the onset of post-operative cerebrovascular accidents including transient or permanent hemiplegia or aphasia. Paralysis involving the ninth to twelfth cranial nerves was also common. Sometimes this was produced by the tumour but often followed surgery (Van Asperen de Boer *et al.*, 1981). For such reasons Lees *et al.* (1981) advocate the advice of an ENT surgeon before surgical treatment of chemodectoma is undertaken. In the elderly, or in those with generalized illness, a conservative approach is indicated for the risk of damage to the carotid arteries is too great and the small risk of malignant change has to be accepted.

Tumours of the other glomera

The other glomera throughout the body may give rise to tumours which have a similar histological picture to that of the chemodectoma in being composed of chief cells. Thus it seems likely that these tumours as a group arise from cells of neurectodermal origin and not from neuroblasts which form the chromaffin and ganglion cells in the sympathetic ganglia (Kjaergaard, 1973). These tumours do not incorporate a significant number of sustentacular cells or nerve endings, thus pointing to their true neoplastic nature. Differences betweeen this group of tumours are the result of their widely differing anatomical sites which result in characteristic clinical pictures.

Glomus jugulare tumour

Glomera located along the course of the tympanic branch of the glossopharyngeal nerve or the circular branch of the vagus nerve may give rise to this tumour of the middle ear. It commonly forms a reddish mass which bleeds easily and appears initially as an aural polyp (Glenner and Grimley, 1974). The jugular tumour may originate laterally in the temporal bone, to erode the floor of the hypotympanum to present as a mass in the middle ear (Hatfield *et al.*, 1972). Occasionally the tumour arises in the adventitia of the jugular bulb (Guild 1941) and presents as a lesion at the base of the skull with enlargement of the jugular foramen and may extend as finger-like projections into the lumen of the jugular vein. The chief cells contain dense-core vesicles and may secrete adrenaline and produce clinical symptoms of phaeochromocytomas. The glomus jugulare tumour is said to be commoner in women.

Laryngeal chemodectoma

This usually arises on either side of the midline above the anterior end of the vocal cords. It may also arise between the thyroid and cricoid cartilages or from glomera within the recurrent branch of the vagus nerve. It commonly leads to pain in the throat, hoarseness and bleeding and has a tendency to become malignant (Vetters and Toner, 1970).

Aortic body tumour

Such a tumour may arise from glomera situated in the adventitia of the pulmonary trunk, ascending aorta and subclavian artery. Usually it is attached to, or lies within, the pericardium surrounding the left auricle or intimately associated with the ascending aorta. Such intimate relation of these tumours to the great vessels frequently precludes resection (Surakiatchanukul *et al.* 1971).

Orbital chemodectoma

Such a tumour may occur at any time between childhood and middle age. There is no sex preponderance. The usual presentation is visual loss with orbital throbbing. If the optic nerve is involved there is also macular degeneration. Glaucoma may be present. This tumour is red-brown to tan in colour, somewhat lobulated and is rubbery on section. It may be as much as 4 cm in diameter and occurs in the retrobulbar area (Thacker and Duckworth, 1969) or involves the rectus muscles (Fisher and Hazard, 1952).

Vagal body tumour

This arises from nests of glomic cells within the perineurium of the vagus nerve just below or at the ganglion nodosum. Frequently the ganglion is completely replaced. There is a sex preponderance weighted towards females as in the glomus jugulare tumour. There is usually a mass in the anterolateral aspect of the neck leading to hoarseness and difficulty in swallowing. The histological features are the same as those found in tumours of other glomera (Fig. 10.8). As with the other glomera, the vagal body tumour may become malignant, with metastases to cervical lymph nodes or bones (Burman, 1955).

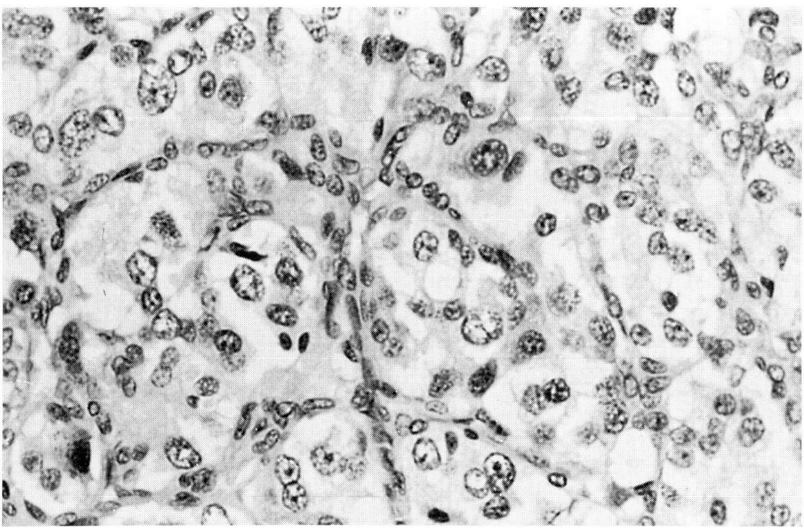

Fig. 10.8 Vagal body tumour from a man of 49 years showing a micro-alveolar pattern. (HE × 375)

Tumour of the organ of Zuckerkandl

This arises from the organ of Zuckerkandl or one of the other retriperitoneal glomera associated with the sympathetic chain at the bifurcation of the abdominal aorta (Attia *et al.*, 1961). It may occur at other sites between the renal vessels and the origin of the iliac arteries. The tumour is ovoid or lobulated, and is tan, grey or red in colour. Such neoplasms may be as large as 15 cm in diameter. It presents as an abdominal mass and may give rise to low back pain. It occurs in a younger age group than that seen in tumours of other glomera. Metastases to regional lymph nodes and the skeleton are not uncommon. A high proportion of these tumours show functional activity due to secretion of catecholamines producing the signs and symptoms of phaeochromocytoma.

Phaeochromocytoma of urinary bladder

This very rare neoplasm appears to arise from small nests of glomic tissue within the trigone and commonly about the ureteric orifices. It will bulge into the bladder leading to painless haematuria.

Pulmonary chemodectoma

The nature of tumours and nodules within the lung resembling glomic tissue is considered in the following chapter.

References

Albores-Saavedra, J. & Durán, M.E. (1968). Association of thyroid carcinoma and chemodectoma. *American Journal of Surgery* **116**, 887.

Alpert, L.I. & Bochetto, J.F. (1974). Carotid body tumor: ultrastructural observations. *Cancer* **34**, 564.

Arias-Stella, J. & Bustos, F. (1976). Chronic hypoxia and chemodectomas in bovines at high altitudes. *Archives of Pathology* **100**, 636.

Attia, R., Golden, R.L. & Ziffer, H. (1961). Nonchromaffin-staining functional tumor of the organs of Zuckerkandl. *New England Journal of Medicine* **264**, 1130.

Barroso-Moguel, R. & Costero, J. (1962). Argentaffin cells of carotid body tumour. *American Journal of Pathology* **41**, 389.

Bensch, K.G., Gordon, G.B. & Miller, L.R. (1965). Electron microscopic and biochemical studies on the bronchial carcinoid tumor. *Cancer* **18**, 592.

Berdal, P., Braaten, M., Cappelen, C. Jnr, Mylius, E.A. & Walaas, O. (1962). Noradrenaline-adrenaline producing nonchromaffin paraganglioma. *Acta Medica Scandinavica* **172**, 249.

Browse, N.L. (1982). Carotid body tumours. *British Medical Journal* **284**, 1507.

Brown, J.W., Burton, R.C. & Dahlin, D.C. (1967). Chemodectoma with skeletal metastasis: Report of two cases. *Mayo Clinic Proceedings* **42**, 551.

Burman, S.O. (1955). The vagal body tumor. *Annals of Surgery* **141**, 488.

Chase, W.H. (1933). Familial and bilateral tumors of the carotid body. *Journal of Pathology and Bacteriology* **36**, 1.

Capella, C. & Solcia, E. (1971). Optical and electron microscopical study of cytoplasmic granules in human carotid body tumours and glomus jugulare tumours. *Virchows Archives, B, Zellpathologie* **7**, 37.

Chedid, A. & Jao, W. (1974). Hereditary tumours of the carotid bodies and chronic obstructive pulmonary disease. *Cancer* **33**, 1635.

Cone, T.E. (1958). Recurrent pheochromocytoma. Report of a case in a previously treated child. *Pediatrics* **21**, 994.

Conley, J.J. (1965). The carotid body tumor — a review of 29 cases. *Archives of Otolaryngology* **81**, 187.

Costero, I. & Barroso-Moguel, R. (1961). Structure of carotid body tumor. *American Journal of Pathology* **38**, 127.

Costero, I. & Chevez, A.Z. (1962). Carotid body tumor in tissue culture. *American Journal of Pathology* **40**, 337.

Cragg, R.W. (1934). Concurrent tumours of the left carotid body and both Zuckerkandl bodies. *Archives of Pathology* **18**, 635.

Donald, R.A. & Crile, G. (1948). Carotid body tumors. *American Journal of Surgery* **75**, 435.

Fanning, J.P., Woods, F.M. & Christian, H.J. (1963). Metastatic carotid body tumor. *Journal of the American Medical Association* **185**, 129.

Fisher, E.R. & Hazard, J.B. (1952). Nonchromaffin paraganglioma of the orbit. *Cancer* **5**, 521.

Fries, J.G. & Chamberlain, J.A. (1968). Extra-adrenal pheochromocytoma *Surgery* **63**, 268.

Glenner, G.G., Crout, J.R. & Roberts, W.C. (1962). A functional carotid-body-like tumor secreting levarterenol. *Archives of pathology* **73**, 230.

Glenner, G.G. & Grimley, P.M. (1974). *Tumors of the extra-adrenal paraganglion system (including chemoreceptors).* Armed Forces Institute of Pathology, Washington.

Grimley, P.M. & Glenner, G.G. (1967). Histology and ultrastructure of carotid body paragangliomas. Comparison with the normal gland *Cancer* **20**, 1473.

Goormaghtigh, N. & Pattyn, S. (1954). A presumably benign tumor and a proved malignant tumor of the carotid body. *American Journal of Pathology* **30**, 679.

Guild, S.R. (1941). A hitherto unrecognised structure, the glomus jugularis, in man. *Anatomical Record* **79**, (Suppl. 2), 28.

Gustilo, R.B., Lober, P.H. & Salavich, E.L. (1965). Chemodectoma (carotid body tumor) metastizing to the bone; case report. *Journal of Bone and Joint Surgery* **47**, 155.

Hamberger, C.A., Hamberger, C.B., Wersäll, J. & Wågermark, J. (1967). Malignant catecholamine — producing tumour of the carotid body. *Acta Pathologica et Microbiologica Scandinavica* **69**, 489.

Hatfield, P.M., Jones, A.E. & Schulz, M.D. (1972). Chemodectomas of the glomus jugulare *Cancer* **30**, 1164.

Javid, H., Chawla, S.K., Dye, W.S., Hunter, J.A., Najafi, H., Goldin, M.D. & Serry, C. (1976). Carotid body tumor. *Archives of Surgery* **111**, 344.

Kahn, L.B. (1976). Vagal body tumor (nonchromaffin paraganglioma, chemodectoma, and carotid body-like tumor) with cervical node metastasis and familial association. Ultrastructural study and review. *Cancer,* **38**, 2367.

Katz, A.D. (1964). Carotid body tumors in a large family group. *American Journal of Surgery* **108**, 570.

Kjaergaard, J. (1973). *Anatomy of the carotid glomus and carotid glomus-like bodies (non-chromaffin paraganglia).* F.A.D.L.'s Forlag Copenhagen.

Lattes, R. (1950). Nonchromaffin paraganglioma of ganglion nodosum carotid body, and aortic arch bodies. *Cancer* **3**, 667.

Le Compte, P.H. (1951). Tumors of the Carotid Body and Related Structures. *Fascicle 16. Atlas of Tumor Pathology.* Armed Forces Institute of Pathology, Washington.

Lees, C.D., Levine, H.L., Beven, E.G. & Tucker, H.M. (1981). Tumors of the carotid body. Experiences with 41 operative cases. *American Journal of Surgery* **142**, 362.

Lewison, E.F. & Weinberg, T. (1950). Carotid body tumors; case report of bilateral carotid body tumors with unusual family incidence. *Surgery* **27**, 437.

Monge, C. (1966). Demografia y Altitud en el Peru. *In: Poblacion y Altitud* Ed: L. Sobrevilla. Imprenta sesator Lima, Peru.

Morfit, H.M., Swan, H. & Taylor, E.R. (1953). Carotid body tumors; report of twelve cases including one case with proven visceral dissemination. *Archives of Surgery* **67**, 194.

Mulligan, R.M. (1950). Chemodectoma in the dog. *American Journal of Pathology* **26**, 680.
McNealy, R.W. & Hedin, R.F. (1939). Surgery of carotid body tumours. *Journal of the International College of Surgeons* **2**, 285.
Pryse-Davies, J., Dawson, I.M.P. & Westbury, G. (1964). Some morphologic, histochemical, and chemical observations on chemodectomas and the normal carotid body, including a study of the chromaffin reaction and possible ganglion cell elements. *Cancer* **17**, 185.
Rabson, A.S. & Elliott, J.L. (1957). Carotid body tumors with regional lymph node involvement with report of a case. *Surgery* **42**, 381.
Reese, H.E. & Bergman, P.A. (1963). Malignant carotid body tumors. *Annals of Surgery* **157**, 232.
Robertson, D.I. & Cooney, T.P. (1980). Malignant carotid body paraganglioma: Light and electron microscopic study of the tumor and its metastases. *Cancer* **46**, 2623.
Romanski, R. (1954). Chemodectoma (non-chromaffinic) paraganglioma of the carotid body with distant metastasis with illustrative case. *American Journal of Pathology* **30**, 1.
Saldaña, M.J. & Salem, L.E. (1970). High altitude hypoxia and chemodectomas. *American Journal of Pathology* **59**, 91*a*.
Saldaña, M.J., Salem, L.E. & Travezan, R. (1973). High altitude hypoxia and chemodectomas. *Human Pathology* **41**, 251.
Shamblin, W.R., ReMine, W.H., Sheps, S.G. & Harrison, E.G. (1971). Carotid body tumor (chemodectoma). Clinicopathologic analysis of ninety cases. *American Journal of Surgery* **122**, 732.
Sprong, D.H. & Kirby, F.G. (1949). Familial carotid body tumors: report of nine cases in 11 siblings. *Annals of Western Medicine and Surgery* **3**, 241.
Staats, E.F., Brown, R.L. & Smith, R.R. (1966). Carotid body tumors, benign and malignant. *Laryngoscope* **76**, 907.
Surakiatchanukul, S., Goodsitt, E. & Storer, J. (1971). Chemodectoma of the aortic body. *Chest* **60**, 464.
Thacker, W.C. & Duckworth, J.K. (1969). Chemodectoma of the orbit. *Cancer* **23**, 1233.
Toker, C. (1967). Ultrastructure of a chemodectoma. *Cancer* **20**, 271.
Turnbull, F.M. (1954). Malignancy in carotid body tumors with presentation of a proved case of metastases to the lungs. *The Western Journal of Surgery, Obstetrics and Gynecology* **62**, 382.
Van Asperen de Boer, F.R.S., Terpstra, J.L. & Vink, M. (1981). Diagnosis, treatment and operative complications of carotid body tumours. *British Journal of Surgery* **68**, 433.
Vetters, J. M. & Toner, P.G. (1970). Chemodectoma of larynx. *Journal of Pathology* **101**, 259.
Westbury, G. (1963). Carotid body tumors. *Current Medicine and Drugs* **4**, 3.
Wilson, H. (1966). Carotid body tumors. *Surgery* **59**, 483.

11. Glomic Tissue and the Pulmonary Circulation

Glomic tissue is associated anatomically with the pulmonary circulation at its most proximal and distal segments. Thus, a glomus is present at the bifurcation of the pulmonary trunk, and microscopic collections of glomic tissue are to be found occasionally around the pulmonary venules in the pulmonary parenchyma. However, as we shall see, the physiological relationship of these tissues to the pulmonary circulation is much less certain.

The 'glomus pulmonale'

Many glomera are present around the heart and great vessels and one of them is present on the dorsal aspect of the bifurcation of the pulmonary trunk. Krahl (1960) found its situation there so constant that he designated it 'the glomus pulmonale' believing it to be the homologue of the carotid body for the sixth branchial arch from which the pulmonary circulation is derived. He found it in the cat, dog, rat, cow, and chimpanzee as well as in man (Krahl, 1962). We sought such a glomus by staining with 1 per cent methylene blue solution the surface of the pulmonary trunk removed at necropsy from a man of 56 years who had died of myocardial ischaemia due to coronary occlusion (Edwards and Heath, 1969). This demonstrated a small plexus of nerves just posterior and caudal to the bifurction. A block of tissue from the wall of the pulmonary trunk was removed from this area and serial sections of it were cut and stained for histological examination. This enabled us to demonstrate with ease glomic tissue in the exact position predicted by Krahl (1962) but the mere situation of a glomus in the wall of the pulmonary trunk does not prove that it is the 'glomus pulmonale' of derivatives of the sixth branchial arch. The crucial point is its source of blood supply. Krahl (1962) believed that this glomus receives its blood supply from the pulmonary trunk but Comroe (1962) found no physiological evidence of a chemoreceptor attached to the pulmonary arteries and responsive to low oxygen tension. He was unable to produce immediate respiratory stimulation by injection into the pulmonary arteries of cyanide, which is a known stimulator of chemoreceptor tissue. Comroe believed that to prove conclusively the existence of a glomus pulmonale which is quite distinct from the aortic body it is essential to demonstrate both glomera in the same subject. One should be able to demonstrate a pulmonary glomus with a blood supply from the pulmonary trunk, and an aortic glomus with a blood supply from the aorta or one of its branches.

Subsequently, we studied the site and blood supply of the mediastinal glomera, including the one on the surface of the pulmonary trunk, in a male 32-week-old stillbirth and in a male child aged 3 years killed in a road traffic accident (Edwards and Heath, 1970). At the same time we carried out confirmatory corrosion cast studies in Wistar albino rats. We found that the intertruncal glomera have a solely systemic arterial blood supply through branches of the coronary arteries and aorta. There is no supply from the pulmonary circulation to support the concept of a 'glomus pulmonale'. Our studies confirmed the observation of Becker (1966) that there is a more or less continuous chain of glomera extending from around the coronary arteries through the intertruncal area of the superior mediastinum to the tissues lying between the arch of the aorta, the right pulmonary artery, and the ductus arteriosus (or ligamentum arteriosum). They also supported his finding that in man and animals these glomera are supplied entirely by systemic arterial blood and largely by intertruncal branches of the coronary arteries.

Perivenous nodules of glomic tissue

When the pathologist examines sections of specimens of lung taken routinely at post-mortem, he will occasionally come across small nodules of tissue around pulmonary venules that have been considered to be glomic in nature. In fresh specimens of lung at necropsy these nodules are firm, greyish-pink and translucent and may bulge above the pleural surface. They are rounded but somewhat irregular and appear encapsulated. They show no evidence of haemorrhage or necrosis. When large numbers of them are present they may give the spurious appearance of miliary tuberculosis. In the case reported by Korn *et al.* (1960) there were several hundreds of these nodules in all lobes, situated mainly in the peripheral portions of the lung. They were often subpleural, especially at the insertions of septa into the pleura, and they were surrounded by much carbon pigment.

Estimations of their prevalence vary somewhat. Thus Korn and his associates found them in 0.3 per cent of necropsies while Spain (1967) found them in as many as 4 per cent. Thurlbeck (1979) believed that they are found in about 0.5 per cent of sections of lung taken for routine necropsy histology but in about 4 per cent of cases when a special, careful search is made for them. Such nodules are small, measuring up to 1.0×0.6 mm in diameter (Edwards and Heath, 1972).

They are located in the interstitium adjacent to and around pulmonary venules (Fig. 11.1). There is an expansion of the septa containing them and fibrous septa radiate irregularly from the central mass where the bulk of the tissue is found. The pulmonary capillaries are stretched over the constituent cells so that the displaced capillary loops separate the cells from the alveolar spaces (Fig. 11.1).

The individual cells have been described as showing a distinct whorling pattern (Kuhn and Askin, 1975) or being arranged in a concentric fashion so that those at the periphery of the nodule are thinner and more elongated than those at

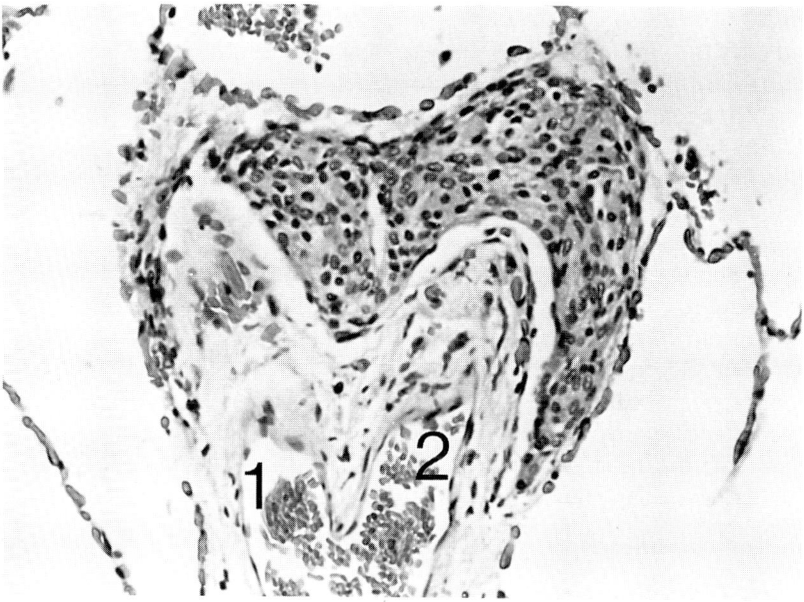

Fig. 11.1 Tangential cut through pulmonary venule formed by two tributaries, 1 and 2, which pass downwards. Enfolding these two tributaries is a roughly crescentic mass of cells which prove to have ultrastructural features similar to those of meningocytes or sustentacular cells. From a man of 57 years with systemic hypertension. (HE × 235)

the centre (Churg and Warnock, 1976). The cells have a round, oval, or elongated nucleus and indistinct cytoplasmic margin. Some of them are large and spindle-shaped or elongated. A few of the nuclei are pyknotic. The cells show neither argentaffinity nor argyrophilia (Churg and Warnock, 1976).

Multiple nodules of this type appear to have first been described by Korn and his associates (1960) who regarded them as multiple small chemodectomas. Other authors are not so certain of their nature and think they may be hamartomatous or even hyperplastic (Spencer, 1962). They must be distinguished from 'tumourlets' (Whitwell, 1955) which are minute proliferations of argyrophilic Feyrter cells arising from small bronchi and bronchioles.

Spain (1967) found a relationship between these perivenous nodules and pulmonary thromboembolism and thought they might represent hyperplasia secondary to ischaemia. Churg and Warnock (1976) noted an association with pulmonary injury, cardiac failure, chronic bronchitis and emphysema, and pulmonary thromboembolism and thought that in some way they were related to alveolar hypoxia. They stated that these nodules are commoner in women.

Ultrastructure

The electron microscopy of these structures has been studied by Kuhn and Askin (1975) and by Churg and Warnock (1976). The former authors found many of the nodules in the right upper lobe of a 69-year-old Negro woman. They found that the constituent cells show several distinct features. They do not contain neurosecretory vesicles, indicating that they are not chief glomic cells. Instead they contain tangled cytoplasmic fibrils 6–10 nm in width (Kuhn and Askin, 1975; Churg and Warnock, 1976). The cells also show multiple processes which show a complex interweaving and interdigitation between cells, so that sometimes only a gap of 20 nm separated cell membranes. Adjacent cells are connected by typical well-formed desmosomes, with associated intra-cytoplasmic fibrils (Kuhn and Askin, 1975; Churg and Warnock, 1976). The cells contain a scattering of mitochondria, a few cisterns of endoplasmic reticulum and a small Golgi apparatus. No axons are present. Many cells have a few lipid or lipofuscin droplets but glycogen is rarely found.

It is clear that these cells do not resemble chief cells or the cell of a chemodectoma which contain neurosecretory vesicles, and which have a basement membrane around epithelial groups, fenestrated endothelium in their capillaries, and many mitochondria and ribosomes. The relation of the nodules to veins is reminiscent of that of arachnoid granulations to cerebral dural sinuses and in fact both Kuhn and Askin (1975) and Churg and Warnock (1976) believe that the cells on ultrastructural grounds are reminiscent of those of a meningioma arising from arachnoid granulations. The tangle of cytoplasmic fibrils and the intimate interdigitation characteristic of the cells is reminiscent of the sustentacular cells of glomic tissue (Chapter 6). It is of interest that Kuhn and Askin (1975) conclude that, since the cells have such little resemblance to chief cells, the nodules they form are not derived from glomic tissue. However, the possibility that the tissue is composed of sustentacular cells has to be considered.

Some of the reported examples of perivenous nodules in the lung occurred in patients with systemic hypertension which is, however, a common condition. In a case that we reported in a woman of 63 years, death was due to pontine haemorrhage secondary to raised blood pressure (Edwards and Heath, 1972). It will be recalled that in Chapter 8 we point out that proliferation of sustentacular cells in the carotid bodies occurs in systemic hypertension.

Pulmonary chemodectoma

The fact that these perivenous nodules are composed of elongated cells reminiscent of sustentacular cells or the cells of arachnoid granulations suggests that they represent a different entity from discrete subpleural tumours of the lung which are large and have the characteristic alveolar pattern of carotid body tumours. Such pulmonary tumours have been reported by a number of authors including Heppleston (1958) and Fawcett and Husband (1967). They form well-encapsulated, sizeable masses just beneath the visceral pleura. Their cut surface is grey and is partially lobulated by septa. Heppleston (1958) reported a chemodectoma in the lung of an achondroplastic dwarf. It formed a friable mass, 4 × 3 × 3 cm, in relation to an interlobar fissure and was encapsulated in fibrous tissue so that it could be easily shelled out after excision of the overlying visceral pleura. Histologically these large subpleural tumours have an alveolar pattern with rounded or polyhedral clear cells arranged in 'zellballen' (Heppleston, 1958) (Chapter 10). The cells have abundant eosinophilic cytoplasm with fine granules and the cell boundaries are not always very distinct so that the cellular tissue presents the appearance of a syncytium. The nuclei are large and vesicular with a fine chromatin pattern and prominent nucleoli and uncommonly they show pleomorphism or giant and multinucleate forms. The significance of this is described in Chapter 10. Reticulin stains reveal the pattern characteristic of chemodectomas.

References

Becker, A.E. (1966). The glomera in the region of the heart and great vessels. A microscopical-anatomical and histochemical study. *M.D. thesis*. Drukkerij Aemstelstad, Amsterdam.

Churg, A.M. & Warnock, M.L. (1976). So-called 'minute pulmonary chemodectoma'. A tumour not related to paragangliomas. *Cancer* **37**, 1759.

Comroe, J.H. (1962). In: *Ciba Foundation Symposium on Pulmonary Structure and Functions* (p. 70) Eds: A.V.S. de Reuck and M. O'Connor.

Edwards, C. & Heath, D. (1969). Microanatomy of glomic tissue of the pulmonary trunk. *Thorax* **24**, 209.

Edwards, C. & Heath, D. (1970). Site and blood supply of the intertruncal glomera. *Cardiovascular Research* **4**, 502.

Edwards, C. & Heath, D. (1972). Pulmonary venous chemoreceptor tissue. *British Journal of Diseases of the Chest* **66**, 96.

Fawcett, F.J. & Husband, E.M. (1967). Chemodectoma of lung. *Journal of Clinical Pathology* **20**, 461.

Heppleston, A.G. (1958). A carotid body-like tumour in the lung. *Journal of Pathology and Bacteriology* **75**, 260.

Korn, D., Bensch, K., Liebow, A.A. & Castleman, B. (1960). Multiple minute pulmonary tumors resembling chemodectomas. *American Journal of Pathology* **37**, 641.

Krahl, V.E. (1962). The glomus pulmonale: its location and microscopic anatomy. In: *Ciba Foundation Symposium on Pulmonary Structure and Function* (p. 53). Eds: A.V.S. de Reuck and M. O'Connor.

Krahl, V.E. (1960). The glomus pulmonale. *Bulletin of the School of Medicine Maryland* **45**, 36.

Kuhn, C. & Askin, F.B. (1975). The fine structure of so-called minute pulmonary chemodectomas. *Human Pathology* **6**, 681.

Spain, D.M. (1967). Intrapulmonary chemodectomas in subjects with organizing pulmonary thromboemboli. *American Review of Respiratory Disease* **96**, 1158.

Spencer, H. (1962). In: *Pathology of the Lung* (pp. 690–92). Pergamon, London.

Thurlbeck, W.M. (1979). Neoplasia of the pulmonary vascular bed. In: *Pulmonary Vascular Disease* (p. 629). Ed. K.M. Moser. Marcel Dekker Inc., New York, Basel.

Whitwell, F. (1955). Tumourlets of the lung. *Journal of Pathology and Bacteriology* **70**, 529.

12. Carotid Sinus

The origin of the internal carotid artery is often dilated and easy to delineate from the portions of the common and internal carotid vessels lying respectively proximal and distal to it (Fig. 1.2). It is termed the carotid sinus and its macroscopic and histological features are consistent with the fact that it has a more complex function than the mere conduction of blood. The carotid sinus is often obvious on naked-eye examination, appearing fusiform or triangular in shape (Fig. 1.2) and commonly extending proximally to involve the bifurcation. It is, however, variable in appearance and may be difficult to distinguish. It is virtually impossible to measure the length of the carotid sinus as its extremities merge imperceptibly into its adjacent vessels. The transverse diameter of the carotid sinus is usually about that of its parent common carotid artery, although it sometimes exceeds it. It is, however, distinctly greater than that of the immediately adjacent and distal internal carotid artery, the narrowing often being abrupt (Table 12.1).

Histological structure

Qualitative and quantitative studies of the histology of the walls of the vessels forming the bifurcation of the common carotid artery (Heath *et al.*, 1973) confirm that the carotid sinus has a specialized structure.

Qualitative histology

The parent vessel of the sinus, the common carotid artery, is an elastic conducting artery with a structure similar to that of the aorta. Its thick media contains many crenated elastic laminae running roughly parallel with one another. The bulk of the media is composed of smooth-muscle fibres with a few collagen fibres but in its outer zone there may be areas where the elastic fibres are crowded together with little or no intervening muscle.

In contrast, in the carotid sinus there is an abrupt thinning of the media (Fig. 12.1). Its inner zone still has the structure of a conducting elastic artery but in the outer zone the elastic fibrils are packed tightly together with no muscle fibres interposed between them. In some subjects the media of the carotid sinus is very thin and composed largely of a compact layer of elastic fibrils. With increasing age the inner portion of the media is fibrous.

Table 12.1 Quantitative histological features of the carotid sinus, and common and internal carotid arteries

Subject	Common Carotid Artery		Carotid Sinus		Internal Carotid Artery	
	Range	*Mean*	*Range*	*Mean*	*Range*	*Mean*
Greatest transverse diameter on fresh specimen (mm)	6.0–9.3	8.0	5.3–9.3	7.6	3.0–4.3	4.7
Greatest transverse diameter on *histological examination (mm)	4.4–7.6	6.4	4.4–7.7	6.3	3.0–5.0	4.0
Absolute medial thickness in μm	626–1034	767	164–588	319	318–590	463
Medial thickness as % of external diameter	8.3–16.7	12.1	2.5–8.7	5.2	10.1–15.8	12.4
Thickness of intimal proliferation as % of external diameter	1.0–9.6	4.5	2.1–19.7	10.0	0–2.4	1.2
Percentage of lumen occluded by atherosclerosis	–	–	12.8–69.0	37.4	–	–

*It will be noted that the external diameters of the fixed arteries as determined by histological measurement are smaller than the transverse diameters measured on fresh specimens. This is because the external diameters measured between diametrically opposite points on the external elastic laminae do not include the adventitia as do measurements on photographic prints of the fresh specimens. Furthermore, histological measurements are made on tissue inevitably shrunken as a result of fixation and processing.

On the distal side of the carotid sinus the internal carotid artery reverts rapidly into the structure of a typical muscular artery in which the media is largely composed of tightly-packed smooth muscle with but few small elastic fibrils. The media of the internal carotid artery is obviously thicker than that of the sinus, although lying distal to it. Its internal elastic lamina is thick and well-defined with elastic fibrils in the subjacent zone of the media. There is a compact zone of tightly packed parallel elastic fibrils in the zone of the demarcation between the outer media and adventitia.

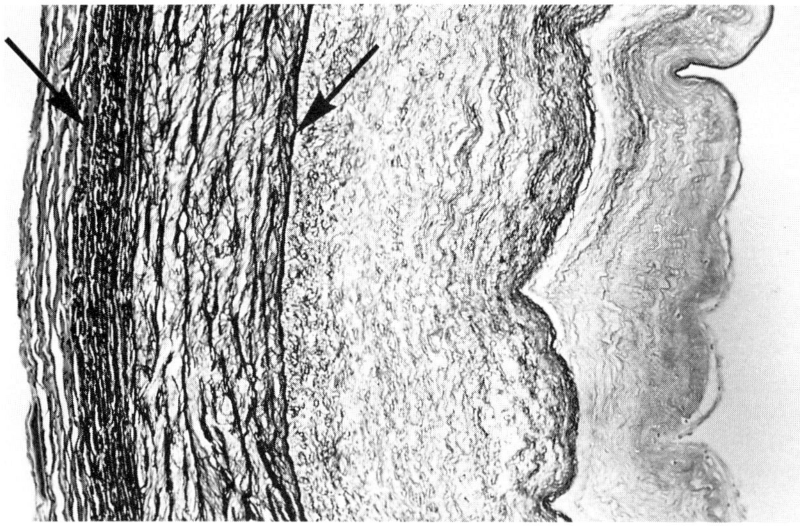

Fig. 12.1 Arc of transverse section of carotid sinus from a man of 61 years. There is a pronounced thinning of the media the limits of which are indicated by arrows. The elastic fibrils in the outer media are tightly packed together. There is severe intimal fibro-elastosis. (EVG × 65)

Quantitative histology

The medial thickness of the carotid sinus is much less than that of the carotid artery on either side of the sinus. The range and mean values of medial thickness expressed in absolute terms and as a percentage of the external diameter of the vessel are shown in Table 12.1. The data confirm that the carotid sinus is a definite anatomical entity characterized by an abrupt thinning of the media which is just as rapidly replaced by the normal muscularity of the media on distal progression in the internal carotid artery (Table. 12.1). In fact the medial thickness of the carotid sinus is only some 5 per cent of the external diameter of the artery, a figure more appropriate to the pulmonary than the systemic circulation.

Age-change and atherosclerosis

Like all blood vessels the carotid sinus is subject to age-change taking the form of proliferation of myofibroblasts in the intima and ending as intimal fibrosis or fibroelastosis. However, although the sinus is a normal anatomical structure, it has the general configuration of a small aneurysm. As such it is subjected to increased haemodynamic stresses that result in exaggerated age-changes and also in the development of atherosclerosis. Thus from the very outset of life it has a form that almost inevitably will lead to pathological changes likely to interfere with its function.

When the carotid sinus is cut open, it commonly shows severe atherosclerosis with degeneration, rigidity and often calcification of much of its wall thickness. There is frequently thickening, puckering and scarring of its lining so that the sinus is contracted. On histological examination the thick layer of intimal atherosclerosis commonly extends into the underlying media, fragmenting its elastic fibrils and leading to a 'moth-eaten appearance' (Fig. 12.2). On transverse

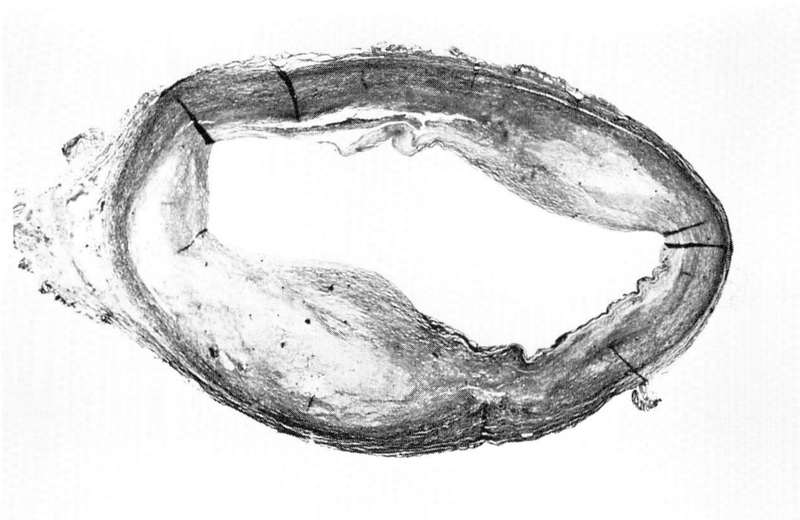

Fig. 12.2 Transverse section of right carotid sinus from a man of 63 years with bronchial carcinoma and duodenal ulcer. It shows severe atherosclerosis leading to an appreciable diminution in the lumen and fibrosis of the media. (EVG × 9)

sections of the carotid sinus from 38 subjects coming to necropsy we measured the areas occupied by the patent lumen (a), intimal proliferation (b) and media (Heath *et al.*, 1973). It thus proved possible to measure the percentage blockage of the lumen of the carotid sinus by intimal proliferation which equals $\frac{b}{a + b} \times 100$ per cent. We found the linear regression equation predicting percentage occlusion from age to be: $0.40 \times \text{age} + 13.0$ ($r = 0.50$; $P < 0.01$). In Table 12.1 the mean values and ranges for percentage occlusion of the carotid sinus by atherosclerosis are shown for the same 13 cases in which the other quantitative histological investigations had been made.

It has been known for many years that the carotid sinus is very prone to the development of atherosclerosis. Keele (1933) found it to be involved in no fewer than 50 of the 55 cases in his series. Samuel (1956) examined the internal carotid arteries in 82 cases and found atheroma in 74 of them, particularly in the sinus and cavernous parts, the petrous and cerebral segments being much less frequently and severely involved. The carotid sinus was atherosclerotic in 60 instances and the process was severe in 15.

The carotid sinus as baroreceptor

More than half a century ago it was shown in animals that pressure on the walls of the carotid sinus leads to slowing of the heart and a fall in systemic blood pressure (Hering, 1927; Heymans, 1929). This would appear to be the physiological function associated with the characteristic thinning of the media of the carotid sinus described above. Such a structure suggests that the sinus might well be more distensible than its neighbouring common and internal carotid arteries to allow stimulation of the branches of the glossopharyngeal nerve and the initiation of baroreceptor reflexes. One suspects that many physiologists, from their experiments on animals, think of the carotid sinus as a thin-walled, highly elastic segment of the carotid arterial bifurcation. However, as we have seen above, the histological adaptation of the wall of the carotid sinus to subserve a baroreceptor rôle is heavily modified by age-change intimal fibrosis and atherosclerosis. Indeed, as we have seen, in the elderly the carotid sinus may become hardly more than a fibrous or even partly calcified sac. For this reason we carried out a study of the extensibility of the carotid sinus (Winson *et al.*, 1974).

Extensibility

We measured the extensibility of the carotid sinus in 30 subjects coming to necropsy between the ages of 16 to 77 years, using the apparatus we had employed previously to measure the extensibility of the pulmonary trunk in cases of congenital heart disease (Harris *et al.*, 1965). This consisted of a central Perspex chamber in which a 1 cm length of circumferential strip of the sinus was stretched between two vertical clamps. The lower one was attached to a platform which could be moved up and down between runners. The upper one was suspended vertically above the lower clamp by means of a stiff steel wire attached to one arm of a balance, the opposite arm of which acted as a pointer against a circular scale which had been previously calibrated between 0 and 100 g weight. Thus by moving the platform up and down the strip of artery could be subjected to increasing extensible loads the magnitude of which could be read from the scale on the balance. The length of the strip at any load was measured by means of a Vernier microscope. In view of the variation in initial length the extension produced by each extensible load was expressed as a percentage of the original unstretched length, given by the formula:

$$\frac{\text{stretched length} - \text{original length}}{\text{original length}} \times 100$$

When the results were expressed graphically it was found that there was a curved relation between extensile load and percentage extension produced by that load, so that with increasing extensile loads the extensibility decreased (Fig. 12.3). This relation is similar to that described previously in systemic arteries elsewhere in the body (Burton, 1954) and in the human pulmonary trunk (Harris *et al.*, 1965). Roach and Burton (1957) ascribed the curved shape of the length-tension diagram of the walls of arteries to the elastic fibres having a shorter relaxed length relative to the collagen fibres. Thus, the first and more horizontal part of the graph was thought to be due to the extension of the elastic fibres alone, and the more vertical part of the graph to gradual recruitment of collagen fibres.

The extensibility of the carotid sinus decreases with age (Fig. 12.3). Thus we found that at an extensile load of 100 g the carotid sinus of a boy of 16 years extended by as much as 64 per cent of its original circumference, whereas in a

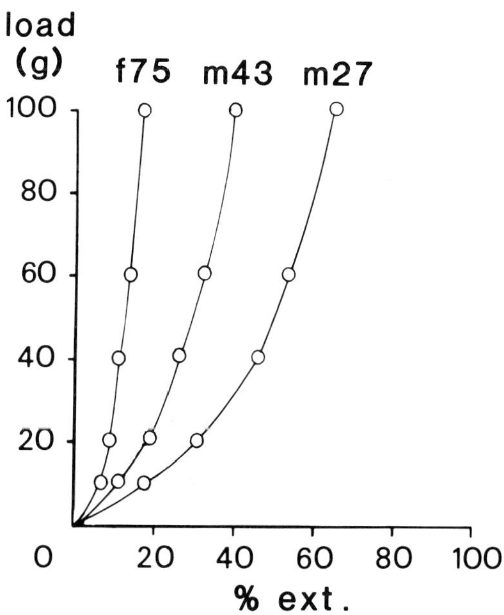

Fig. 12.3 Circumferential extensibility of the right carotid sinus (*open circles*) in two men aged 43 and 27 years old and in a woman aged 75 years. The extensibility falls progressively with age.

woman of 75 years it extended by only 16 per cent. Such a fall in extensibility has been previously described in both systemic and pulmonary arteries (Burton 1954; Harris *et al.*, 1965) and is almost certainly attributable to the increase of collagen within the arterial walls. In the case of the carotid sinus the loss of circumferential extensibility is certainly due to the pronounced age-change intimal fibroelastosis and atherosclerosis described above.

As a result of its predilection to age-change intimal fibrosis and atherosclerosis the carotid sinus is more extensible than the common carotid artery only in the very young and at loads below 40 g. From early adulthood onwards and with greater loads it is less extensible (Fig. 12.4).

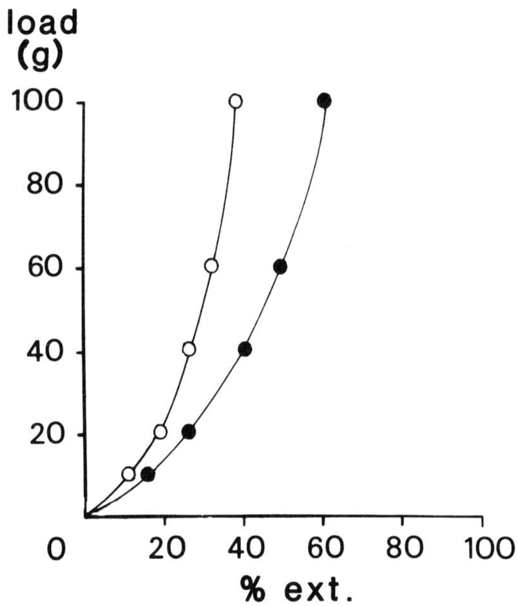

Fig. 12.4 Circumferential extensibility of the right carotid sinus (*open circles*) and right common carotid artery (*closed circles*) in a 43-year-old man. The carotid sinus is less extensible than the common carotid artery.

Baroreflex insensitivity

Clinical physiologists have confirmed that the loss of arterial distensibility which occurs both in ageing and in systemic hypertension reduces the efficiency of the carotid sinus. Gribbin and his associates (1971) studied baroreflex sensitivity in 61 male and 20 female patients, aged 19–66 years, whose mean systemic arterial pressure ranged from 70 to 150 mmHg. The index of sensitivity they used was the increase in pulse interval in milliseconds which occurs reflexly in response to each mmHg rise in systolic pressure induced by the intravenous injection of phenylephrine. They found that increasing age and systemic arterial pressure act independently to reduce baroreflex sensitivity. Sleight (1971) found that a linear relation is obtained when the systolic pressure of a pulse beat is plotted against the pulse interval that follows. Thus the slope of this line may be employed as an index of the baroreflex arc. He thought that increased intravascular pressure may inactivate the baroreceptors by damaging the nerve endings or splint them in the stiff, fibrous walls of the sinus. The effects of atherosclerosis on baroreflex sensitivity must depend to some extent on the orientation of the receptors in the arterial wall. If these are pulled circumferentially then an increased rigidity of the arterial wall should lead to a decreased baroreceptor response. If, on the other hand, they are compressed from within outwards, an increased rigidity of the vessel wall may not have such an effect. It is known that digital compression of a stiff carotid sinus will still stimulate receptors.

Carotid sinus syndrome

Weiss and Baker (1933) suggested that occasionally the reflexes arising in the carotid sinus in man are abnormally sensitive and may be responsible for attacks of unconsciousness and convulsions. They showed that such attacks could be induced by pressure over one carotid sinus. The cause of syncope was considered to be cerebral anoxaemia resulting from cardiac asystole or a sudden fall in systemic blood pressure. This clinical syndrome was described in further detail in a subsequent paper by Weiss and his colleagues in 1936. They were convinced that a wide variety of signs and symptoms may result from this so-called carotid sinus syndrome. These included fainting, dizziness and weakness, hyperpnoea, facial pallor, bradycardia, numbness and tingling of the extremities, convulsions and drowsiness. Short attacks of syncope may develop when the patient is in the upright position. They found that the syndrome involved middle-aged and elderly subjects in whom there is likely to be atherosclerosis of the carotid sinus with rigidity and diminished extensibility of its walls. Mechanical stimulation of the carotid sinus does not give rise to symptoms in young subjects and increasing pressure in the sinus leads only to a slight and temporary fall in systemic blood pressure. However, stimulation of the diseased carotid sinus in the middle-aged or elderly may induce symptoms as well as a characteristic fall in blood pressure. Weiss and his colleagues were so convinced of the validity of the syndrome as a clinical entity that they recognized three types; the vagal, the depressor, and the cerebral.

Further cases of the syndrome were but rarely reported until Morley *et al.* (1982) described no fewer than 70 patients who had been treated by artificial pacing over a period of four years. Leatham (1982) found this wealth of cases so surprising that he felt it raised the whole issue of the definition of the carotid sinus syndrome. Leatham thought that reflex slowing of sinoatrial rate from carotid sinus massage was an almost universal finding and that it was more pronounced in 'older subjects' (undefined) and was more noticeable in patients with disease of the conducting tissue. He thought that cardiac slowing in the cases reported by Morley and his colleagues might be primarily sinoatrial disease rather than an abnormality of the wall of the carotid sinus. Leatham did not accept as valid the statement that none of their patients had overt sick sinus syndrome on the resting or 24 hour electrocardiogram, because he feels that patients with episodes of even extreme bradycardia may have weeks or even months of normality. Thus, Leatham concluded that most, if not all, of the patients described by Morley and his colleagues had sinoatrial disease. He felt that further work was required to decide whether primary carotid sinus syncope is other than an extremely rare medical curiosity. He regarded carotid sinus stimulation more as a means of unmasking conduction disease.

References

Burton, A.C. (1954). Relation of structure to function of the tissues of the wall of blood vessels. *Physiological Reviews* **34**, 619.

Gribbin, B., Pickering, T.G., Sleight, P. & Peto, R. (1971). Effect of age and high blood pressure on baroreflex sensitivity in man. *Circulation Research* **29**, 424.

Harris, P., Heath, D. & Apostolopoulos, A. (1965). Extensibility of the human pulmonary trunk. *British Heart Journal* **27**, 651.

Heath, D., Smith, P., Harris, P. & Winson, M. (1973). The atherosclerotic human carotid sinus. *Journal of Pathology* **110**, 49.

Hering, H.E. (1927). *Die Karotissinusreflexe auf Herz und Gefässe.* Theodor Steinkopff, Dresden.

Heymans, C. (1929). *Le sinus carotidien et les autres zones vasosensibles réflexogènes.* Presses Universitaires de France, Paris.

Keele, C.A. (1933) Pathological changes in the carotid sinus and their relation to hypertension. *Quarterly Journal of Medicine n.s.* **2**, 213.

Leatham, A. (1982) Carotid sinus syncope. *British Heart Journal* **47**, 409.

Morley, C.A. , Perrins, E.J., Grant, P., Chan, S.L., McBrien, D.J. & Sutton, R. (1982). Carotid sinus syncope treated by pacing. Analysis of persistent symptoms and role of atrioventricular sequential pacing. *British Heart Journal* **47**, 411.

Roach, M.R. & Burton, A.C. (1957). The reason for the shape of the distensibility curves of arteries. *Canadian Journal of Biochemistry and Physiology* **35**, 681.

Samuel, K.C. (1956) Atherosclerosis and occlusion of the internal carotid artery. *Journal of Pathology and and Bacteriology* **71**, 391.

Sleight, P. (1971). What is hypertension? Recent studies in neurogenic hypertension. *British Heart Journal* **33** (Suppl.), 109.

Weiss, S. & Baker, J.P. (1933). The carotid sinus reflex in health and disease: its role in the causation of fainting and convulsions. *Medicine* **12**, 297.

Weiss, S., Capps, R.B., Ferris, E.B. Jnr & Munro, D. (1936). Syncope and convulsions due to a hyperactive carotid sinus reflex. *Archives of Internal Medicine* **58**, 407.

Winson, M., Heath, D. & Smith, P. (1974). Extensibility of the human carotid sinus. *Cardiovascular Research* **8**, 58.

Index

Page numbers set in italic denote the position in the text of illustrative material.